Telemedicine for Adolescent and Young Adult Health Care

Yolanda N. Evans • Sarah A. Golub
Gina M. Sequeira

Editors

Telemedicine for Adolescent and Young Adult Health Care

A Case-based Guide

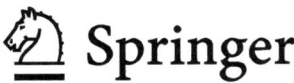 Springer

Editors
Yolanda N. Evans
University of Washington
Seattle, WA, USA

Sarah A. Golub
University of Washington
Seattle, WA, USA

Gina M. Sequeira
University of Washington
Seattle, WA, USA

ISBN 978-3-031-55759-0   ISBN 978-3-031-55760-6   (eBook)
https://doi.org/10.1007/978-3-031-55760-6

This Springer imprint is published by the registered company Springer Nature Switzerland AG
The registered company address is: Gewerbestrasse 11, 6330 Cham, Switzerland

Paper in this product is recyclable.

Contents

Chapter 1
A General Overview of Telehealth in Pediatrics

Mark D. Lo

Virtual healthcare has finally "come of age" for the pediatric population, especially for the adolescent patient. It took a pandemic to accelerate widespread acceptance and adoption [1], but now telehealth is a legitimate care modality in healthcare systems. Policies and legislation continue to be created to accommodate this modality [2], yet the result remains that access to care is broadened beyond the four walls of a physical building, and virtual care can now be in almost any location with almost anyone participating.

Overview of Telehealth and Definitions

With new technologies and care modalities come new definitions. Although the terms "telehealth" and "telemedicine" are closely related, we use the definition of telehealth as a broader umbrella term, under which telemedicine resides [3]. Telemedicine is the live, synchronous communication between provider and patient using digital or telecommunication platforms. Most often, we think of videoconferencing platforms on computer or mobile devices using the Internet as telemedicine. But there is increasing interest and adoption of "audio-only telemedicine" which often takes places over the phone and is useful for specific clinical scenarios such as

---

Audience: primary care clinicians, adolescent medicine specialists (including dieticians, psychologists, social workers, school-based providers), and all healthcare clinicians supporting adolescents through telehealth.

M. D. Lo (✉)
University of Washington School of Medicine, Seattle, WA, USA

Telehealth and Digital Health, Seattle Children's, Seattle, WA, USA
e-mail: Mark.lo@seattlechildrens.org

© The Author(s), under exclusive license to Springer Nature Switzerland AG 2024
Y. N. Evans et al. (eds.), *Telemedicine for Adolescent and Young Adult Health Care*, https://doi.org/10.1007/978-3-031-55760-6_1

1

in the adolescent population where the provider and patient are having a conversation about the patient's health and the adolescent patient cannot find Internet access or a private space without others looking at their screen or may only have access to a landline phone.

Telehealth, the broader definition, includes more than telemedicine [4]. Telehealth can be defined as any healthcare delivered virtually to the patient by a remote provider, outside of the four walls of the healthcare facility [5]. Notably, it also includes asynchronous care modalities, often referred to "store-and-forward." This is the remote diagnostic interpretation of patient data by a provider with intent to deliver care to that patient and not in real-time. An example of this would be a teen patient who sends a photo of a concerning rash to the dermatology specialist, who will respond with care recommendations and/or diagnosis at a later time based on that photo, but the provider will not directly speak to the patient. Another example of asynchronous telehealth might be remote patient monitoring (RPM) by data collection, as in a continuous glucose monitor that a diabetic patient is wearing. That data is collected and often synchronized to a format in the digital cloud that a provider can download, view, and monitor in order to make specific care recommendations for that patient.

Telehealth also may include health educational webinars where patients can learn about their condition or care recommendations as part of a group setting. These videoconferences may be live or recorded and may be specific or generic to the condition or patient. Examples in pediatrics might be educational webinars on topics such as "Introduction to Autism" or "Going Through Puberty." Various videoconference platforms make it possible for patients and families to submit questions to webinar panel members, chat with others in the videoconference for advice, or break out into smaller virtual "rooms" for more specific attention or conversation. Finally, the definition of telehealth can also be extended to include "mHealth": mobile device apps and wearable devices that are directed toward the health of the patient. Apps can be recommended, or "prescribed" to patients by providers for such purposes including caloric/dietary monitoring, mental health improvements or meditation, or recording exercise and heart rates.

History of Telehealth for Pediatrics and Associated Barriers

Pediatric medicine has historically trailed adult medicine in therapies and innovations, and telehealth is no different. Barriers to provider adoption of telehealth for both pediatric and adult populations have generally focused on lack of payment, lack of technology or training, and uncertainty around regulation and licensure [6]. Despite American Association of Pediatrics recommendations for acceptance and adoption of telehealth, most primary care pediatricians did not embrace this care modality largely due to insufficient payment [7].

When telehealth was not a necessary care modality, most primary care pediatricians, schools, and adolescent medicine specialists were not adopting it. The lack of payment and lack of familiarity with pediatric telehealth made it that much more jarring when virtual care became a necessity during the COVID-19 pandemic.

Pandemic Response and Aftermath

It is impossible to discuss pediatric telehealth without referencing the role that the COVID-19 pandemic has played in changing provider and patient perspectives on telehealth. The stay-at-home notices, school and work closures, and community lockdowns all forced healthcare providers to pivot to any means necessary to deliver care remotely to their patients. This took the form of phone calls, video conferences, text chats, and emails. Legislation, payors, and healthcare policies all had to quickly adapt to a virtual care model. Waivers and policy exceptions made it possible for healthcare to continue to be delivered, sometimes with greater access or convenience for patients. The fact that healthcare could no longer be delivered in person greatly accelerated the adoption of telehealth, and this was occurring in parallel with the educational system, social meetings, and relationships all converting to the virtual space.

As infection rates fluctuate and policymakers strive to clarify what a post-pandemic and post-public health emergency landscape will look like, it remains to be determined how prominent a place pediatric telehealth will occupy in healthcare. Adolescents may have their own sense of whether they prefer in-person or virtual visits; they are a population that may be more at ease with switching between the two visit types. However, the adolescent telehealth experience may be limited in what kinds of medical concerns may be addressed during the virtual visit, and in-person visits may be better for certain concerns [8, 9]. Various economic and access forces may push for a return to in-person healthcare as the standard, but virtual care has established its foothold in mainstream consciousness. Most healthcare systems understand that a virtual option must be included as a legitimate post-pandemic care modality and should be expected to account for a sizeable percentage of total patient visits.

Digital Health Equity for Pediatric Patients

One significant outcome of the widespread push for telehealth during the pandemic was the confirmation that not all patients had the same access to virtual care. Access to telehealth was different based on race/ethnicity, language of preference, and payment modality, among other factors [10]. This inequity is independent of whether the patient populations are adult or pediatric [11, 12]. Although telehealth is seen as generally improving access by removing geographical barriers, it is limiting access if the patients do not have the means to use the telehealth modality. Multiple areas of inequity have been identified and are especially relevant to the adolescent and pediatric populations: lack of Internet/network bandwidth, lack of devices and technology, lack of digital health literacy/navigation, and lack of trust in the healthcare system [13]. When facilitating virtual visits with adolescents and pediatric patients, opportunities may arise when in partnership with the virtual educational system, since this population are also students and may be able to leverage similar solutions and remedies to bridge the digital education gap. Adolescents already are a vulnerable patient cohort because they do not have full decision-making power over their own healthcare, and digital health inequities add to their vulnerability. It remains very important to consider the additional digital health inequities to this population when proposing telehealth care.

Unique Pediatric/Adolescent Considerations for Telehealth

Although many of the mechanics of telehealth are consistent between adult and pediatric patients, there are several unique characteristics of the pediatric and adolescent telehealth experience (Table 1.1). These characteristics must be taken into account whenever virtual care is established for patients who are not yet adults. Pediatric/adolescent telehealth is largely impacted by the fact that the patient is usually not the primary decision-maker for their own health, and navigating this legal reality is important in establishing and continuing virtual care.

Consent

The role of the adult family member/guardian/parent in establishing telehealth care for the adolescent or pediatric patient must always be addressed. Adolescents are still minors and are not yet in total control of their own health decisions. As such, virtual visits must confirm parental or guardian consent in order to proceed. This can be done verbally and documented by provider or can be a physical signature of the parent/guardian. Similar to consenting adults for telehealth, important aspects of obtaining consent for pediatric virtual care include the offering of an in-person visit

Table 1.1 Unique characteristics of the adolescent and pediatric telehealth visit

Consent required (with state-specific consent waivers for adolescents)	May have restricted access to technology
Familiarity with technology and socialized to technology ("digital native")	Privacy is not guaranteed
School attendance as a possible telehealth location	Adolescents and pediatric patients should not submit to physical exam of sensitive areas online
Pediatric special needs require access to pediatric-specific expertise and therapies	Greater impact of health maintenance to long-term health

Source Dr. Mark Lo

option if desired (although the patient will have to travel), the recognition of lack of an in-person physical examination, the recognition of technology limitations or potential interruptions, and establishing contact info should the visit be interrupted or an emergency arise. Certain states have different exceptions around adolescents being allowed to consent for their own telehealth care without approval or notification of a parent/guardian. These exceptions largely center on emancipated minor status, reproductive health, mental health, and substance abuse chief complaints.

Technology

The use of technology for telehealth is a unique but mixed issue for adolescent patients. Adolescents are some of the most savvy users of technology compared to any age cohort, able to flexibly adapt to different interfaces, devices, and platforms. They are socialized to technology and can easily communicate with each other via mobile device, chat groups, videoconference, asynchronous image or video sharing, text, etc. From one perspective, this "digital native" status makes them an ideal candidate group for telehealth since digital navigation may not be as much of a hindrance to them as compared to other age groups. Conversely, the adolescent cohort may not have the same access to technology and devices that adults have, thus limiting telehealth as a viable care modality for this group. Parental/guardian-enforced limitations on screen time and physical control of those devices may also limit access to telehealth for the adolescent age group. Adolescents may also need to rely on others for high-speed Internet, charging battery, etc., and their potential lack of access to technology must be considered when offering them virtual visits.

Privacy

Similarly, adolescent and pediatric patients may not have control of their physical environment to ensure a private, secure location in which to participate in a telehealth visit. If confidential information is being discussed, teens may not feel that their home location or environment is truly private from listening ears. Headphones may help, but the teen patient may not be comfortable participating in a virtual visit if they do not want their parent/guardian to be hearing what they are saying. There have also been questions around information technology (IT) security and the aspect of having uninvited people barging into telehealth sessions because they had an access hyperlink or meeting ID. It is vital to ensure that telehealth visits are locked down from an IT security standpoint and only invited individuals are able to access the virtual visit. In the same content area of privacy and security, adolescents and pediatric patients should not submit to virtual physical exams that require them to expose parts of their body to an online camera, especially sensitive areas. For younger patients there may be a concern about normalizing the exposure of sensitive areas to camera for a remote audience. If the physical exam part of a visit requires examination of a sensitive area, the virtual visit may not be best option for an adolescent or pediatric patient and an alternative in-person visit should be pursued.

School Setting

Most adolescent and pediatric patients are unique in the fact that they attend full-time school during the day. Unlike the workplace, schools generally have an embedded health maintenance and management component through school nurses or infirmaries/sick rooms. School nurses may triage ill children, deliver medications, or hold students out of class while recovering from injury. These are settings for private, individualized medical care that can be applied to telehealth as well. School telehealth visits are an effective method of delivering virtual healthcare to adolescent or pediatric patients. Several school telehealth programs have been successful in reducing missed school for the patient and missed work for the parent/guardian and improving quality of care [14, 15]. If the adolescent patient is unable to secure private space or technology access at home, school may be a viable location where the patient can receive virtual care. Additionally, for those adolescents who are in homeschool or alternative schooling environments, special attention must be given to their ability to access healthcare via technology, and accommodation of their needs must be considered.

Greater Importance of Health Maintenance

Just as regular exercise and activity for children have important ramifications for their later adult physical and mental health [16, 17], the importance of regular monitoring and health maintenance has outsized impact on the long-term health of the pediatric and adolescent patient. Any irregularity identified with subsequent early intervention will have greater impact on the long-term health of the patient, compared to adults. Telehealth is an ideal care modality for checking in with adolescent patients and monitoring ongoing health needs. It eliminates the geography and waiting of in-person visits and can be brief but effective. Screening tools, surveys, and other data intake instruments can be administered over telehealth and can be valuable in identifying any health issues on a regular basis with early identification and intervention. These early interventions are crucial in areas like developmental pediatrics for diagnosis and treatment, behavioral health, therapies such as speech/language, physical therapy, and occupational therapy. Telehealth may also enable quicker access to surgical specialties to identify any medical complaints that surgery may resolve and not have longstanding impact.

Pediatrics as a Specialty

There is an oft-repeated saying in medicine that "Children are not just small adults," used to describe the need for and value of specialized pediatric medicine experts to take care of pediatric patients, versus generalist providers. General practitioners, family medicine providers, and even general emergency medicine providers may not be as comfortable with the vast range of medical, health, behavioral, and social concerns that fall into the pediatric and adolescent age range. The pediatric and adolescent physiology, development, and behavior may be different enough from adults so as to require providers with more pediatric patient experience. Vital signs and "normal patient findings" are unique to the pediatric and adolescent age ranges and are treated differently than adults. Increasing complexity in children with genetic, biochemical, or mitochondrial disorders also requires more expertise and experience, as do the increasing number of extremely premature babies undergoing neonatal resuscitation who might have lingering medical needs or technology dependence. Pediatric-specific behavior health issues such as autism or developmental delay also require expert management. Access to these pediatric specialties such as adolescent medicine or child psychiatry, or access to pediatric services such as feeding or speech therapy may all be significantly improved via telehealth. The wait times for in-person visits may be prolonged, and the specific care needed may not be able to be supplemented with providers who primarily treat adult patients. There often is discomfort by those providers in managing pediatric or adolescent problems, and they would defer to the pediatric specialists for definitive care. Telehealth enables this care to take place in a more timely and effective manner.

The Future of Telehealth in Pediatrics and Adolescent Medicine

Virtual visits with pediatric and adolescent patients have become the norm for many healthcare providers. The frequency of these visits will likely wax and wane over time, but it is doubtful that they will ever completely disappear, now that the value has been established during a global pandemic. The future of telehealth in this patient population will continue to adapt as technology, access, and digital health equity shifts over time. Telehealth as a broader term will include more than synchronous telemedicine videoconferencing. Remote patient monitoring via wearables or Internet-of-things devices will provide distant evaluation, especially in the home setting. The "hospital at home" movement may allow patients to be cared for virtually in their own homes via these technology solutions. Digital health mobile applications that allow patient self-monitoring, reporting, and even self-diagnosing will continue to gain traction. As more healthcare data for pediatric and adolescent patients is stored, deidentified, and manipulated, there will be novel predictive and analytical algorithms based on machine learning (colloquially known as "artificial intelligence") which will be clinically useful in augmenting health management. In the pediatric and adolescent age cohort, gamification for health purposes may incentivize patients via video games to exercise, undergo therapy, or have behavioral and mental health interventions. The "metaverse" continues to develop in the virtual reality and augmented/mixed reality areas, and telehealth of the future may be more immersive and synchronous as it utilizes all the advantages of that space.

Telehealth for pediatric and adolescent patients has been established as a reliable and effective care modality, and the future will bring with it increased ability for remote healthcare providers and patients to connect virtually in order to improve health quality and outcomes for this population.

References

1. Mann DM, Chen J, Chunara R, Testa PA, Nov O. COVID-19 transforms health care through telemedicine: evidence from the field. J Am Med Inform Assoc. 2020;27(7):1132–5.
2. https://telehealth.hhs.gov/providers/policy-changes-during-the-covid-19-public-health-emergency/. Accessed September 21, 2022.
3. https://www.cchpca.org/what-is-telehealth/. Accessed September 21, 2022.
4. https://catalyst.nejm.org/doi/full/10.1056/CAT.18.0268. Accessed September 21, 2022.
5. Telehealth for providers: what you need to know: from coverage to care. U.S. Department of Health and Human Services, revision date March 2021, Publication #12121. https://www.cms.gov/files/document/telehealth-toolkit-providers.pdf accessed September 21, 2022.
6. Olson CA, McSwain SD, Curfman AL, Chuo J. The current pediatric telehealth landscape. Pediatrics. 2018;141(3):e20172334.
7. Sisk B, Alexander J, Bodnar C, Curfman A, Garber K, McSwain SD, Perrin JM. Pediatrician attitudes toward and experiences with telehealth use: results from a national survey. Acad Pediatr. 2020;20(5):628–35.
8. Barney A, Buckelew S, Mesheriakova V, Raymond-Flesch M. The COVID-19 pandemic and rapid implementation of adolescent and young adult telemedicine: challenges and opportunities for innovation. J Adolesc Health. 2020;67(2):164–71.
9. Qiu Y, Coulson S, McIntyre CW, Wile B, Filler G. Adolescent and caregiver attitudes towards telemedicine use in pediatric nephrology. BMC Health Serv Res. 2021;21(1):537. Published 2021 Jun 1
10. Nouri SS, Khoong EC, Lyles CR, Karliner LS. Addressing equity in telemedicine for chronic disease management during the Covid-19 pandemic. NEJM Catalyst. 2020;1–13. https://doi.org/10.1056/CAT.20.0123.
11. Curfman A, McSwain SD, Chuo J, et al. Pediatric telehealth in the COVID-19 pandemic era and beyond. Pediatrics. 2021;148(3):e2020047795.
12. Katzow MW, Steinway C, Jan S. Telemedicine and health disparities during COVID-19. Pediatrics. 2020;146(2):e20201586.
13. Sieck CJ, Sheon A, Ancker JS, Castek J, Callahan B, Siefer A. Digital inclusion as a social determinant of health. NPJ Digit Med. 2021;4(1):52.
14. North S, Dooley DG. School-based health care. Prim Care. 2020;47(2):231–40.
15. Williams S, Xie L, Hill K, et al. Potential utility of school-based telehealth in the era of COVID-19. J Sch Health. 2021;91(7):550–4.
16. Boreham C, Riddoch C. The physical activity, fitness and health of children. J Sports Sci. 2001;19(12):915–29.
17. Rodriguez-Ayllon M, Cadenas-Sánchez C, Estévez-López F, et al. Role of physical activity and sedentary behavior in the mental health of preschoolers, children and adolescents: a systematic review and meta-analysis. Sports Med. 2019;49(9):1383–410.

Chapter 2
Telehealth for Adolescents: Confidentiality Protections and Challenges

Abigail English and Lisa K. Mihaly

Introduction

Increased availability and use of telehealth has expanded accessibility of essential health-care services for adolescents and young adults [1–4]. The expansion of telehealth offers promising potential for specific populations of young people whose access is especially limited; these may include, for varied reasons, rural youth, those in state custody (foster care or juvenile justice), youth with chronic Illness or disability, young people experiencing homelessness, LGBTQ and BIPOC youth, and others who have been historically marginalized [5]. At the same time, assuring protection for adolescents' privacy and the confidentiality of their health information presents challenges in the telehealth arena that encompass key clinical and legal considerations.

In this chapter, the term "telehealth" refers to clinical care and not to other uses of telehealth services, such as health education and public health activities. For clinical purposes, telehealth services may be conducted in a variety of ways, including telephone or audio-video technology, and on different electronic platforms, such as a patient portal or Zoom. In this chapter, "privacy" refers to a patient's interest in controlling access to information about themselves and their health, and "confidentiality" refers to the protection of their health information based on ethical

A. English (✉)
Center for Adolescent Health & the Law, Chapel Hill, NC, USA

Gillings School of Global Public Health, University of North Carolina at Chapel Hill, Chapel Hill, NC, USA

L. K. Mihaly
Department of Family Health Care Nursing/School of Nursing, Division of Adolescent Medicine/School of Medicine, University of California San Francisco, San Francisco, CA, USA
e-mail: lisa.mihaly@ucsf.edu

9

principles and legal requirements, although these terms are sometimes used interchangeably in clinical settings and the professional literature. In addition, the term "adolescent" has no fixed legal definition; in this chapter, the term "adolescent" is used to refer both to those under age 18 years who are legally minors and those age 18 years or older who are legally adults in most US jurisdictions. When referring to those who are legally minors, the term "adolescent minor" is used.

Several important questions for telehealth visits are:

- Who is authorized to consent to the visit and the care provided?
- Whose consent is required for telehealth services?
- What privacy concerns exist?
- How can the confidentiality of adolescents' electronic health information (EHI) be protected?

These questions are important whenever health care is provided to adolescents, but the answers may vary or entail special considerations when services are delivered via telehealth.

In considering these questions, it is important to note that adolescents often consult with and share information with their parents when making health-care decisions; they also do so with other trusted adults. Ensuring that confidentiality protections are available when needed is not designed to inhibit voluntary communication and sharing of information between adolescents of any age and their parents. Clinicians are well-positioned to assist adolescents in sharing information with their parents when legally necessary or clinically appropriate, and parents are well-positioned to support and advise their adolescent children. However, not all adolescents have supportive parents and some adolescents, at specific times, have particularly sensitive concerns they need to share with a health-care professional and prefer to keep private. Decades of research findings have documented the impact of privacy concerns on adolescents' access to and use of health-care services as well as the role of health-care providers and parents in relation to confidentiality protection [6]. These considerations are relevant in the telehealth arena as well as for in-person care.

The policy and technology landscape—both for telehealth and for the delivery of adolescent health services—is evolving in ways that have implications for protecting the confidentiality of adolescents' health information. For instance, restrictions on access to reproductive health services and care for transgender adolescents have major impacts: the recent US Supreme Court decision removing federal constitutional protection for abortion and policy actions at the state level related to gender-affirming health care have generated heightened concerns about threats to adolescents' privacy [7, 8]. The availability of adequate insurance coverage for telehealth visits is essential but not assured; also, communications related to health insurance claims give rise to specific confidentiality considerations. Laws requiring increased access to and interoperability of EHI make the need for methods of granular segmentation and patient control of EHI increasingly urgent; granular segmentation refers to the use of technology to identify separate elements of a patient's information that can then be appropriately shared or protected from sharing consistent with ethical and legal requirements. The technology required for tele-health visits and the varied access to technology among adolescents limits the extent to which some adolescents can benefit from telehealth (see Chap. 3 on health equity). These issues all raise serious equity concerns.

Consent for Telehealth Services

Consent requirements for adolescent telehealth visits may have privacy and confidentiality implications. If the consent of someone other than the adolescent patient is required, the fact of the visit is not confidential, although some information about it may be protected. The impact of consent requirements on confidentiality concerns will vary depending on the reason for the visit, the relationship between the adolescent and the parent or other person such as a legal guardian or other adult custodian, and the laws that apply where the visit takes place. A clinical scenario and several variations highlight the context in which consent requirements may—or may not—have confidentiality implications.

- Scenario 1. CC is a 16 year old scheduled for a telephone visit to discuss back pain she has had for the past few days. At the beginning of the phone call, the provider obtains her consent for the telephone visit. A few minutes later, her father takes the phone from her and tells the provider he thinks a telephone visit is inappropriate for her concerns.

  - Variation 1a. Patient consents to a telephone visit for abdominal pain. Provider is worried about pelvic inflammatory disease (PID) and refers the patient to the emergency department (ED), which contacts parents to obtain consent for further treatment. Parents are angry they were not involved in decision about ED visit.
  - Variation 1b. Patient wants to be seen in-person for abdominal pain. Patient is worried about sexually transmitted infection (STI) but the family does not know that. Parent consents only to a video visit rather than an in-person visit because of COVID concerns.
  - Variation 1c. Patient consents to a telephone visit to authorize a refill of her oral contraceptive pills (OCP), which the family knows she is taking for dysmenorrhea.
  - Variation 1d. Patient wants to obtain a refill of her OCP via a telehealth visit by telephone. Her parents do not know she is taking OCPs. During the call, her mother takes the phone and demands to know the purpose of the visit.

Scenario 1 and each of the variations illustrate the questions of who is authorized to consent and whose consent is required. Specifically, is it sufficient for the patient to consent or is the consent of a parent, guardian, or other adult required? An overarching question is whether the fact that these are telehealth visits, either by telephone or audio-video technology, requires any additional or different consent than would be required for an in-person visit for any of these purposes. Beyond this overarching question, an important factor in determining the consent requirements is whether the visit is for care that the patient is authorized to consent for independently, which may vary depending on where she lives.

In Scenario 1, the patient is an adolescent minor who is being seen for a primary care concern—back pain—that would ordinarily require parental consent. The fact that the visit is a telehealth visit conducted over the telephone would not eliminate the need for consent from an authorized person (which might be the patient or the parent depending on the specific situation), so the father's apparent withdrawal of consent may be significant. In each of the variations, issues related to STIs or OCPs are involved, so the patient may be legally allowed to consent on her own, but the question remains as to whether the use of telehealth has any significance with respect to consent. In variation 1b, consent is not a barrier; the patient could have consented for an in-person visit related to STI diagnosis, and the father has given consent for a video telehealth visit. When a telehealth visit leads to other care, such as an ED visit in Variation 1a, costs and insurance coverage issues may lead to loss of confidentiality even if the care, such as for PID, might be something for which the adolescent could consent.

From a clinical and ethical perspective, for Scenario 1 and each of the variations, several considerations are relevant in relation to obtaining consent for the visit. Because the process of obtaining the parent's consent results in disclosure of the fact the visit is occurring, it is important for the provider to be aware in advance whether this would create any difficulty for the patient. Thus, the nature of the patient's relationship with her parents; the sensitivity of the reason for the visit; the extent to which the patient has already, or is willing to, share sensitive information with her parents and her reasons for doing so or not; and the specific legal requirements for consent are all important factors.

Legal Framework

To understand the legal framework that applies to consent for a telehealth visit, it is important to know the age of the patient, the specific reason for the visit, and the services that will be provided. Because laws determining consent for adolescents' health care as well as legal requirements for telehealth consent vary from state to state, it is also necessary to consider where the adolescent is located and where the services are provided. Delivery of services interstate raises complex issues that arose frequently during the COVID pandemic but are beyond the scope of this chapter [9, 10]. It is important for health-care providers to obtain current legal advice on their own state laws governing consent and telehealth.

There is no fixed legal definition of "adolescent." Some young people who are referred to as adolescents, and receive care from adolescent health professionals, are age 18 or older and are legally adults in most US jurisdictions. These young adults are legally allowed to consent for their own health care, which would include consenting for telehealth visits. Adolescents who are younger than age 18 are legally minors, and specific consent requirements apply to their care, which may involve obtaining parental consent or the consent of another adult who has the legal authority to make medical decisions for them or may allow them to consent for their own care. Every state has laws that allow adolescents to consent for their own care in certain circumstances. These "minor consent laws" are based either on the specific status or living circumstances of the adolescent minor or on the services they are seeking [11–13] (see Box 1).

Box 1 Minor Consent Laws

Minors who may consent to all or most health care[a]	Services for which some or all minors may consent[a]
Emancipated minor	Contraceptive care
Minor living apart from parents	Pregnancy-related care
Minor older than a specific age	Abortion
"Mature" minor	STI prevention, diagnosis, or treatment[b]
Married minor	Infectious/reportable disease prevention,
Minor parent	diagnosis, or treatment
Minor on active military duty	HIV/AIDS prevention, testing, or treatment
Minor in law enforcement custody	Substance use counseling or treatment
	Outpatient mental health services
	Sexual assault care

[a]These laws vary from state to state. Not every state has laws covering all categories.
[b]Some states use the term sexually transmitted infection (ST); others use venereal disease (VD) or sexually transmitted disease (STD)

As listed in Box 1, in every state, some adolescent minors are allowed to consent for all (or almost all) of their own health care, with wide variation among states. For each group, state law may include age restrictions or other specific criteria. For instance, mature minors must have the capacity for informed consent; minors living apart from their parents may include youth experiencing homelessness but may have to demonstrate financial independence; and the age at which a few states allow minors to consent for all or most of their own care, based specifically on their age, varies from 14 to 16 years.

Also listed in Box 1 are specific services for which adolescent minors may be allowed to consent for themselves. Again, these laws vary from state to state. For instance, some states allow adolescent minors to consent for prevention of STIs or reportable diseases, whereas others limit their consent to diagnosis and treatment. The minor consent services covered by the most state laws are STI care; substance use counseling and treatment; and outpatient mental health services. It is noteworthy that although only two-thirds of states explicitly authorize adolescent minors to consent for contraception, in almost every state minors currently can receive family planning services, including contraception, based on their own consent at sites funded by the federal Title X Family Planning Program [14]. The specific factors—such as age, scope of service, and type of professional authorized to provide the care—vary both among states and even within states depending on the specific service.

One health care service that has been subject to very specific restrictions on access by adolescent minors is abortion [15]. These restrictions are evolving at a rapid pace. For several decades, most states have required parental consent or notification with the alternative option of a judicial bypass proceeding that may enable a minor to obtain an abortion without involving their parents. Those laws may change as abortion is banned or severely limited in an increasing number of states following the recent removal of federal constitutional protection by the US Supreme Court in June 2022, leaving to Congress and states the determination of whether to ban or further restrict abortion or expand protections [16–18]. Health-care providers who offer abortion services, including providing medication abortion via telehealth, must obtain current legal advice about all applicable laws pertaining to abortion, including laws in the state where they practice and where the patient is located, as well as any federal laws related to interstate issues [19].

Beyond the minor consent laws, the question arises as to whether an adolescent who is legally allowed to consent for a health-care service is also authorized to consent when the service is provided via telehealth. This question has two parts. First, does a law that authorizes a minor to consent for care based on their status or the specific service extend to telehealth services? Second, if specific consent is required by state or federal law for telehealth services, is a minor able to give that consent if they are otherwise authorized to consent for the care? In addition to its minor consent laws, every state has one or more laws that create specific requirements for telehealth; some of these laws include consent provisions [20, 21]. The application of specific telehealth consent laws to a situation when an adolescent minor is consenting independently and does not want the fact of the visit shared with parents would require careful analysis based on a state's laws that is beyond the scope of this chapter. Current legal advice should be sought if there is uncertainty about specific situations.

Privacy Concerns for Telehealth Visits

When adolescents receive care via telehealth, either as a telephone or audio-video technology visit, significant privacy concerns arise. These concerns are real whether the adolescent is a minor or a young adult. Privacy concerns are most pressing in situations involving sensitive issues such as STI, pregnancy, substance use, mental health, sexual orientation, and gender identity (SOGI) but may extend to any care when an adolescent feels more comfortable sharing a full history with their provider if they can do so without being overheard or seen by others while doing so. In this context, privacy concerns may extend not just to parents but other family members and people within earshot or view. These privacy concerns have been documented in decades of research findings that have shown clearly that adolescents value private communication with their providers [6]. A clinical scenario and several variations highlight the ways in which privacy concerns arise during telehealth visits and possible approaches for mitigating them.

- Scenario 2. PC is a 15-year-old patient who scheduled a video visit to discuss his need for STI screening. He scheduled the appointment himself. He lives with his parents and siblings in a small two-bedroom apartment, where conversations can be heard throughout most of the apartment. His parents are not aware that he has had sex. He is worried that they will kick him out of the house if they find out. PC scheduled the appointment for a time when he thought everyone else in his family would be out of the house. A few minutes after the visit starts, he realizes that his father has come home and can probably hear everything he is saying.

  - Variation 2a. After patient realizes his father is in the house, he switches to texting with his provider rather than speaking out loud. He does not realize that his parents have guessed his password and can access his phone without his knowing.
  - Variation 2b. During the telehealth visit, PC's parents overheard that he had been sexually active with male partners and were threatening to make him engage in therapy to abandon his gay "lifestyle." He left home and was staying either at friends' houses or in a shelter.

Maintaining the physical and electronic privacy of telehealth visits can be a major challenge for patients of any age. Many homes do not have private spaces where an adolescent can engage in a visit without being overheard or seen. Some telehealth visits involve sharing images of sensitive areas of the body that particularly require privacy. Often the patient may be aware that the visit is not private, but the provider will not know this unless they ask specific questions, particularly if parents or other people are in the room or in earshot but off camera. Adolescents use varied strategies for increasing privacy protection, such as sitting in the bathroom with water running to cover sounds or taking calls while working, walking outside, or sitting in a car. Some privacy concerns are specific to a patient's need to shield information from parents, as in Scenario 2 and Variation 2a, while other situations, such as when PC is experiencing homelessness, may not involve parents directly but present significant obstacles to privacy because the patient is outdoors or in a space that is controlled by or accessible to others.

With the increased use of telehealth for adolescents during the COVID-19 pandemic, professional organizations and health-care organizations have developed guidelines and recommendations for how to protect the privacy needed for telehealth visits. For instance, the American Medical Association developed an extensive Telehealth Implementation Playbook, which includes as one of numerous resources a "Telehealth Visit Etiquette Checklist" that mentions privacy as a key element [22]. Some health-care organizations and federally supported Centers of Excellence have also developed useful resources to help providers and patients overcome the privacy challenges [23]. An additional consideration is that sometimes being able to protect a patient's privacy will depend not only on the availability of a private physical space but also on the patient's access to appropriate technology. Some electronic platforms offer greater privacy protections than others and not all patients have the technology they need to use them effectively. Many health systems restrict telehealth visits to a specific platform that is available via their patient portal; independent practitioners may use a variety of platforms. Ensuring that the platforms used offer privacy protection while being accessible to patients are essential considerations. Both the lack of private spaces and the disparities in access to technology raise significant equity concerns (see Chap. 3 on health equity).

Legal Framework

The legal framework that exists to protect privacy for telehealth visits is essentially the same as the framework for health-care visits generally. The array of federal and state health-care privacy laws that protect adolescents when they receive health care in person also applies when they engage in telehealth visits. What has varied, at least during the COVID-19 pandemic, is that enforcement of some of these laws, particularly the HIPAA Privacy Rule and some state privacy laws, were loosened to facilitate a wider range of options for delivering health care via telehealth.

For the past two decades, the HIPAA Privacy Rule has established in federal law a floor of privacy protection; states can provide greater protection but not less. The HIPAA Privacy Rule protects adolescents, including both adolescent minors and those who are young adults [24]. The rule includes many detailed requirements that are beyond the scope of this chapter to enumerate and that are explained extensively elsewhere.

Noteworthy in the present evolution of telehealth service delivery is that the federal agency responsible for enforcement of the HIPAA Privacy Rule, the Office of Civil Rights (OCR) in the Department of Health and Human Services (HHS), issued guidance early in the COVID-19 pandemic directing that "breaches of the HIPAA Privacy and Security Rules that occur in the course of good faith provision of telehealth services will not be subject to enforcement." [25, 26]. This guidance provided much greater latitude to health-care systems and providers in delivering telehealth services than would otherwise have been impossible to implement as quickly as was necessary during the pandemic. This HHS "enforcement discretion" was not extended once the Public Health Emergency (PHE) declaration that was in place throughout the pandemic was lifted in 2023 [26]. In addition, the Notice of Enforcement Discretion issued by HHS applies specifically to the HIPAA Privacy and Security Rules and not to the federal substance use disorder confidentiality regulations known as "Part 2"; similar guidance was issued by the Substance Abuse and Mental Health Services Administration regarding enforcement of the Part 2 rules [27]. Several states have also loosened specific privacy requirements for telehealth visits during the pandemic; the fate of those state policies following the end of the COVID Public Health Emergency ends is not yet clear [20].

In addition to the guidance on Enforcement Discretion, HHS has issued other guidance as well. For instance, HHS states:

> Providers should always use private locations and patients should not receive telehealth services in public or semi-public settings, absent patient consent or exigent circumstances. If telehealth cannot be provided in a private setting, covered health care providers should continue to implement reasonable HIPAA safeguards to limit incidental uses or disclosures of protected health information (PHI). Such reasonable precautions could include using lowered voices, not using speakerphone, or recommending that the patient move to a reasonable distance from others when discussing PHI [28].

Although these recommendations are designed to protect patients' privacy, from a practical perspective, they may not be realistic for many adolescents to implement when engaging in telehealth visits. Nevertheless, providers should be conscious of these factors when conducting telehealth visits with adolescents and should make maximum efforts to determine the degree of privacy available for each visit and tailor communications to ensure that sensitive information is not inadvertently disclosed, taking into consideration the privacy measures the patient is, or is not, able to implement.

HHS also specified which communication platforms were permissible to use during the Public Health Emergency (PHE). As listed in Box 2, approved platforms include only non-public-facing remote communication products; disallowed platforms include public-facing remote communication products.

Box 2 Platforms Approved by HHS for Telehealth Use During the Public Health Emergency

Non-public-facing remote communication products[a]	Public-facing remote communication products[b]
Apple FaceTime	TikTok
Facebook Messenger video chat	Facebook Live
Google Hangouts video	Twitch
WhatsApp video chat	Public chat rooms
Skype	
Zoom	

Source: HHS, Notification of Enforcement Discretion [29]
[a]Platforms approved by HHS for telehealth use
[b]Platforms not approved by HHS for telehealth use

Clinicians who care for adolescents have noted that an adolescent's use of the products that HHS deems permissible may be easily tracked by a parent who has technology skills. Thus, again it is important for providers to be aware of the degree of privacy that can be expected for specific telehealth visits with individual adolescent patients and tailor the verbal and video communications to honor the privacy needs and expectations of their patients. Clinicians may also consult with patients to develop strategies for dealing with concerns about parental tracking.

Following the expiration of the Public Health Emergency, the Enforcement Discretion issued during the COVID-19 pandemic has expired [26]. Therefore, it is now essential for providers to use HIPAA compliant technology for telehealth visits.

Confidentiality of Electronic Health Information

Protecting the confidentiality of electronic health information (EHI) has been an ongoing challenge throughout the years in which electronic records and patient portals have been implemented by health-care systems and providers. Specific challenges for adolescent patients have long been recognized, and myriad efforts have been made to address them. Recently, with the advent of OpenNotes and implementation of the "information-blocking" regulations under the Twenty-first Century Cures Act, the challenges have intensified because much more information is shared and the sharing occurs more quickly than in the past. More frequent use of telehealth to deliver care has not altered the overall framework for confidentiality protection of electronic information but has added new practical and logistical considerations. A clinical scenario and variations highlight some of the challenges in protecting confidentiality of EHI arising from adolescent telehealth visits while complying with applicable legal requirements.

- Scenario 3. EC is a 17 year old who has scheduled a follow-up video visit with her provider. She discusses her interest in the HPV vaccine and plans a follow-up clinic visit to receive the immunization. Her grandparents, who are her guardians, do not want her to receive this vaccine as they believe it will lead to irresponsible sexual behavior. After the visit, the EHR makes the visit notes, immunization records, and scheduled appointment visible in the patient portal, and her grandparents find out about her plans.

  - Variation 3a. During the follow-up video visit, the provider informs the patient of the results of her recent chlamydia test, which was positive. They discuss the treatment needed and how the patient will access the prescription, which her grandparents learn about via phone notifications from the pharmacy to the family's home number.
  - Variation 3b. During the follow-up video visit, the patient requests a renewal of her prescription for anti-anxiety medication. Patient's grandparents had consented to her taking the medication but thought it was for a limited time period when the patient was worried about exams and college applications.

The confidentiality concerns presented by Scenario 3 and its variations are typical ones in adolescent health care and are not limited to the telehealth context. Some adolescents attend virtual visits with their parents or other adult guardians; others do so alone. When an adolescent participates in a telehealth visit without a parent or guardian and wants information associated with the visit to remain confidential, some additional issues arise beyond the typical ones for in-person visits. With visits being scheduled in the patient portal and the patient appearing to be alone during the video visit, the provider may not know the extent to which the patient's parents or guardians are aware of her interactions with her provider. Clarity of communication about this between provider and patient is therefore essential.

This scenario and the variations also offer reminders that consent requirements and confidentiality protections are intertwined. Whether patient lives in a jurisdiction where she is allowed to consent for HPV vaccination has a direct bearing on the significance of whether her related EHI is or is not accessible to her guardians. In Variation 3a, the patient would be able to consent for treatment of chlamydia, but information about the prescription might become known to her grandparents via the patient portal or a phone call from the pharmacy. In Variation 3b, patient's grandparents had consented for her to receive the anti-anxiety medication, but tensions might arise if they learn of her extended use via the portal or the pharmacy. All these situations need to be addressed clinically between the provider and patient, keeping in mind that numerous laws have an impact on how EHI is handled.

Legal Framework

Protecting the confidentiality of adolescents' EHI requires analysis and understanding of the intersection of numerous federal and state laws. This can be especially challenging in the context of telehealth visits, which involve some new or less familiar uses of existing platforms, such as the patient portal.

Major federal laws that have long protected confidentiality of health information, including EHI, are the HIPAA Privacy and Security Rules [30], "Part 2" substance use disorder confidentiality regulations [31], Title X Family Planning Program confidentiality regulations [32], confidentiality regulations for FQHCs [33], confidentiality rules for the Ryan White HIV program [34], and Medicaid's confidentiality requirements [35]. In addition to the federal laws, every state has some laws that affect the confidentiality of health information, including EHI. Most important among these state laws are the confidentiality provisions in state minor consent laws, the general state medical privacy laws, and confidentiality requirements related to specific services such as sexual and reproductive health, HIV, mental health, and substance use. Although these federal and state laws are numerous, deficiencies have been identified in the extent to which they provide adequate protection for individuals' privacy when engaging in telehealth [36].

Along with these federal and state laws, the recent "information blocking" rule under the Twenty-first Century Cures Act is hugely important for EHI confidentiality generally as well as for EHI related to a telehealth visit [37]. Implemented in 2021, the Cures Act's ban on information blocking requires that patients have "immediate access" to their EHI; as of October 2022, the scope of EHI required to be shared increased [38, 39]. The information-blocking rule has resulted in a wide range of information from the EHR being moved very rapidly into the patient portal, where both the patient and any proxies may access it. The shared EHI has included many types of information such as clinician notes, diagnoses, medications, laboratory results, treatment plans, after visit summaries, and any other information included in a patient's medical records. Disclosures also may occur via billing, insurance communications, appointment reminders, medical records requests, and other means.

Although some exceptions—such as for infeasibility, privacy, and preventing harm—are built into the information-blocking rule, the challenges of complying with the regulation have occasioned major concerns among adolescent health-care providers [40–43]. Telehealth by definition involves EHI; therefore, Cures Act compliance for information connected to telehealth visits may especially challenging. The compliance strategies adopted by adolescent health and medicine programs have varied widely, particularly with respect to management of access to the patient portal [44]. The development of granular segmentation capabilities in the EHR is an ongoing process that ultimately may facilitate protection of confidentiality protection for adolescents' EHI [43].

Policy, Technology, and Equity

Ultimately, the most effective approaches for protecting adolescents' EHI related to telehealth visits will require strategies that involve both policy and technology. Equitable access to telehealth for adolescents will also depend on policy and technology solutions.

The policy landscape for telehealth has undergone rapid changes and is continuing to do so. A series of legal and policy changes were implemented to facilitate delivery of telehealth services during the COVID-19 pandemic. These included the issuance of HHS guidance on "Enforcement Discretion" for breaches of the HIPAA Privacy and Security Rules associated with delivery of telehealth services as well as the expanded coverage of telehealth visits in Medicaid, Medicare, and private insurance. These policy developments have changed and are continuing to evolve following the lifting of the COVID Public Health Emergency in ways of importance in the continued use of telehealth.

Not only have policies specific to telehealth been evolving in ways that are important for maintaining adolescents' access to these services, other policies with major implications for the health care of adolescents will affect the confidentiality of adolescents' EHI when they receive care via telehealth. These include the recent reversal of Roe v. Wade and implementation of old and new bans and restrictions on abortion in many states as well as expansion of protection for reproductive rights in others [16–19, 45]; recent bans and restrictions on gender affirming care [46]; and changes to the HIPAA Privacy Rule [47] and to the federal Part 2 substance use disorder confidentiality regulations [48], which could have an impact on the confidentiality of reproductive health and substance use services as well as other care. With each of these legal and policy developments, the potential exists for "surveillance" of adolescents' EHI either by government officials or unauthorized civilians, thereby underscoring the importance of both policies and cyber-security measures to protect against such intrusions. In addition to the harms that are threatened by online surveillance of adolescents, intrusions into the private realms of the provider-patient relationship carry threats for providers as well.

Alongside essential policy protections, key changes in technology are essential for enabling the confidentiality protections that are necessary for appropriate care of adolescents. Technological solutions that allow for granular segmentation of adolescents' EHI data must be found, enabling specific EHI data elements to be treated differently so that some can be shared while others remain private. This is needed to enable compliance with the Twenty-first Century Cures Act information-blocking ban. It is also a critical element in making possible the sharing of information that can improve adolescents' care while identifying and protecting sensitive information that could cause harm if shared. Increasing the control adolescent patients and their providers have over their information can contribute to optimal confidentiality protection that does not conflict with supportive engagement with parents and other providers.

Ultimately, protecting adolescents' privacy and the confidentiality of their health information in the telehealth arena will depend on ensuring that equitable approaches are pursued for all major issues in the realms of policy and technology. Major equity gaps currently exist that undermine privacy and limit confidentiality protections. Many adolescents do not have access to private spaces for telehealth visits. Digital literacy is essential for effective use of telehealth but lags among some young people. Access to technology is widely variable both in terms of devices and Internet access in ways that depend on cost as well as infrastructure. All these factors affect some adolescents more than others: youth of color, adolescents with disabilities and/or complex medical conditions, adolescents in families with lower incomes, marginalized groups such as LGBTQ adolescents, immigrants, youth in state custody, and young people experiencing homelessness are all at greater risk of having their access to telehealth constrained. Without equitable access, equitable protection of privacy and confidentiality is not possible.

References

1. Wood SM, White K, Peebles R, et al. Outcomes of a rapid adolescent telehealth scale-up during the COVID-19 pandemic. J Adolesc Health. 2020;67:172–8. https://doi.org/10.1016/j.jadohealth.2020.05.025.
2. Barney A, Buckelew S, Mesheriakova V, Raymond-Flesch M. The COVID-19 pandemic and rapid implementation of adolescent and young adult telemedicine: challenges and opportunities for innovation. J Adolesc Health. 2020;67:164–71. https://doi.org/10.1016/j.jadohealth.2020.05.006.
3. North S. Telemedicine in the time of COVID and beyond. J Adolesc Health. 2020;67:145–6. https://doi.org/10.1016/j.jadohealth.2020.05.024.
4. Evans YN, Golub S, Sequeira GM, et al. Using telemedicine to reach adolescents during the COVID-19 pandemic. J Adolesc Health. 2020;67:469–71. https://doi.org/10.1016/j.jadohealth.2020.07.015.
5. Ortega G, Rodriguez JA, Maurer LR, Emily E, Witt EE, Perez N, Reich A, Bates DW. Telemedicine, COVID-19, and disparities: policy implications. Health Policy Technol. 2020;9(3):368–71. https://doi.org/10.1016/j.hlpt.2020.08.001.

6. English A 25 Years of Confidentiality Studies—A Bibliography (Appendix G). In: Adolescent & Young Adults Health Care in Minnesota: A Guide to Understanding Consent & Confidentiality Laws. Adolescent & Young Adult Health National Resource Center; and Center for Adolescent Health & the Law; 2019. Available at: http://nahic.ucsf.edu/resource_center/confidentiality-guides/. Accessed 22 Mar 2023.

7. Ralph L, Hasselbacher L. Adolescents and abortion restrictions: disproportionate burdens and critical warnings. J Adol Health 2023;73:221–223. https://doi.org/10.1016/j.jadohealth.2023.05.002. Accessed 27 Dec 2023.

8. Hughes LD, Kidd KM, Gamarel KE, et al. "These laws will be devastating": provider perspectives on legislation banning gender-affirming care for transgender adolescents. J Adolesc Health. 2021;69:976–82. https://doi.org/10.1016/j.jadohealth.2021.08.020.

9. U.S. Department of Health and Human Services. Telehealth licensing requirements and interstate compacts. https://telehealth.hhs.gov/providers/policy-changes-during-the-covid-19-public-health-emergency/telehealth-licensing-requirements-and-interstate-compacts/. Accessed 22 Mar 2023.

10. Center for Connected Health Policy. Cross-state licensing. https://www.cchpca.org/topic/cross-state-licensing-professional-requirements/. Accessed 22 Mar 2023.

11. English A, Bass L, Boyle A, Eshragh F. State minor consent laws: A summary. 3rd ed. Center for Adolescent Health & the Law; 2010. https://www.freelists.org/archives/hilac/02-2014/pdfRo8tw89mb.pdf. Accessed 22 Mar 2023

12. Sharko M, Jameson R, Ancker JS, Krams L, Webber EC, Rosenbloom ST. State-by-state variability in adolescent privacy laws. Pediatrics. 2022;149(6):e2021053458. https://doi.org/10.1542/peds.2021-053458.

13. Guttmacher Institute. An overview of consent to reproductive health services by young people. 2023. Available at: https://www.guttmacher.org/state-policy/explore/overview-minors-consent-law. Accessed 22 Mar 2023.

14. 42 C.F.R. § 51.10.

15. Guttmacher Institute. Parental involvement in minors' abortions. February 2023. Available at: https://www.guttmacher.org/state-policy/explore/parental-involvement-minors-abortions. Accessed 22 Mar 2023.

16. Dobbs v. Jackson Women's Health Org., __U.S.__, 142 S.Ct. 2228 (2022).

17. Guttmacher Institute. Interactive map: US abortion policies and access after Roe. 2023. Available at: https://states.guttmacher.org/policies/. Accessed 22 Mar 2023.

18. Center for Reproductive Rights. After Roe fell: abortion laws by state. Available at: https://reproductiverights.org/maps/abortion-laws-by-state/. Accessed 22 Mar 2023.

19. Sobol L, Ramaswamy A, Salganicoff A. The intersection of state and federal policies on access to medication abortion via telehealth. February 7, 2022. Available at: https://www.kff.org/womens-health-policy/issue-brief/the-intersection-of-state-and-federal-policies-on-access-to-medication-abortion-via-telehealth/. Accessed 22 Mar 2023.

20. Wiegel G, Ramaswamy A, Sobel L, Salganicoff A, Cubanski J, Freed M. Opportunities and barriers for telemedicine in the U.S. during the COVID-19 emergency and beyond. May 11, 2020. Available at: https://www.kff.org/womens-health-policy/issue-brief/opportunities-and-barriers-for-telemedicine-in-the-u-s-during-the-covid-19-emergency-and-beyond/. Accessed 22 Mar 2023.

21. Center for Connected Health Policy. Consent requirements. Available at: https://www.cchpca.org/topic/consent-requirements-medicaid-medicare/. Accessed 22 Mar 2023.

22. American Medical Association. Telehealth implementation playbook. Appendix G.4: Telehealth visit etiquette checklist. 2022. Available at: https://www.ama-assn.org/system/files/ama-telehealth-playbook.pdf. Accessed 22 Mar 2023.

23. The Center of Excellence for Protected Health Information. Telehealth resources. n.d.. Available at: https://coephi.org/?s=telehealth. Accessed 22 Mar 2023.

24. English A, Ford CA. The HIPAA privacy rule and adolescents: legal questions and clinical challenges. Perspect Sex Reprod Health. 2004;36(2):80–6.

25. Office for Civil Rights, U.S. Department of Health and Human Services. FAQs on Telehealth and HIPAA during the COVID-19 nationwide public health emergency. Available at: https://www.hhs.gov/sites/default/files/telehealth-faqs-508.pdf. Accessed 22 Mar 2023.
26. U.S. Department of Health and Human Services. Notice of expiration of certain notifications of enforcement discretion issued in response to the COVID-19 nationwide public health emergency . 88 Fed. Reg. 22380. April 13, 2023. Available at: https://www.govinfo.gov/content/pkg/FR-2023-04-13/pdf/2023-07824.pdf. Accessed 27 December 2023.
27. Substance Abuse and Mental Health Services Administration. COVID-19 public health emergency response and 42 CFR Part 2 guidance. Available at: https://www.samhsa.gov/sites/default/files/covid-19-42-cfr-part-2-guidance-03192020.pdf. Accessed 22 Mar 2023.
28. Office for Civil Rights, U.S. Department of Health and Human Services, Where can providers conduct telehealth? Available at: https://www.hhs.gov/hipaa/for-professionals/faq/3021/where-can-health-care-providers-conduct-telehealth/index.html. Accessed 22 Mar 2023.
29. Office for Civil Rights, U.S. Department of Health and Human Services. Notification of Enforcement Discretion for Telehealth Remote Communications During the COVID-19 Nationwide Public Health Emergency. Available at: https://www.hhs.gov/hipaa/for-professionals/special-topics/emergency-preparedness/notification-enforcement-discretiontelehealth/index.html. Accessed 22 Mar 2023.
30. U.S. Department of Health and Human Services, Summary of the HIPAA Privacy Rule. Available at: https://www.hhs.gov/hipaa/for-professionals/privacy/laws-regulations/index.html. Accessed 22 Mar 2023.
31. 42 C.F.R. Part 2.
32. 42 C.F.R. §59.10.
33. 42 U.S.C. § 254b(k)(3)(C).
34. 42 U.S.C. §§ 300ff-61 and 300ff-62.
35. 42 U.S.C. §§ 1396a(a)(7), 1396d(a)(4)(C).
36. Hale TM, Kvedar JC. Privacy and security concerns in telehealth. AMA J Ethics. 2014;16(12):981–5. https://journalofethics.ama-assn.org/article/privacy-and-security-concerns-telehealth/2014-12. Accessed 22 Mar 2023
37. U.S. Department of Health and Human Services. 21st century cures act: interoperability, information blocking, and the ONC Health IT Certification Program. 85 Fed. Reg. 2562, May 1, 2020. Available at: https://www.govinfo.gov/content/pkg/FR-2020-05-01/pdf/2020-07419.pdf. Accessed 22 Mar 2023.
38. 45 C.F.R. § 171.102.
39. U.S. Department of Health and Human Services. Information blocking: eight regulatory reminders for October 6th. Health IT Buzz. September 30, 2022. Available at: https://www.healthit.gov/buzz-blog/information-blocking/information-blocking-eightregulatory-reminders-for-october-6th. Accessed 22 Mar 2023.
40. The Office of the National Coordinator for Health Information Technology. Cures Act Final Rule: information blocking exceptions. Available at: https://www.healthit.gov/sites/default/files/cures/2020-03/InformationBlockingExceptions.pdf. Accessed 22 Mar 2023.
41. Carlson J, Goldstein R, Hoover K, Tyson N. NASPAG/SAHM statement: the 21st century cures act and adolescent confidentiality. J Adolesc Health. 2021;68:426–8. https://doi.org/10.1016/j.jadohealth.2020.10.020.
42. Bourgeois FC, DesRoches CM, Bell SK. Ethical challenges raised by OpenNotes for pediatric and adolescent patients. Pediatrics. 2018;141(6):e20172745. https://doi.org/10.1542/peds.2017-2745.
43. Pasternak RH, Alderman EM, English A. The 21st century cures act and the ONC Rule: implications for adolescent care and confidentiality protections. Pediatrics 2023 Apr 1;151(Suppl 1):e2022057267K. https://doi.org/10.1542/peds.2022-057267K.
44. Ford CA, Bourgeois F, Buckelew SM, et al. Twenty-first century cures act final rule and adolescent health care: leadership education in adolescent health (LEAH) program experiences. J Adolesc Health. 2021;69(6):873–7. https://doi.org/10.1016/j.jadohealth.2021.09.006.

45. Clayton EW, Embí PJ, Malin BA. Dobbs and the future of health data privacy for patients and healthcare organizations. J Am Med Inform Assoc. 2022 [published online ahead of print, 2022 Sep 1] [published correction appears in J Am Med Inform Assoc. 2022 Oct 04;]; https://doi.org/10.1093/jamia/ocac155.
46. Dawson L, Kates J, Musumeci M. Youth access to gender affirming care: the federal and state policy landscape. June 1, 2022. Available at: https://www.kff.org/other/issue-brief/youth-access-to-gender-affirming-care-the-federal-and-state-policy-landscape/.
47. U.S. Department of Health and Human Services. HIPAA privacy rule to support reproductive health care privacy. 89 Fed. Reg. 32976, Apr. 26, 2024. https://www.govinfo.gov/content/pkg/FR-2024-04-26/pdf/2024-08503.pdf. Accessed 29 Apr 2024.
48. U.S. Department of Health and Human Services. Confidentiality of substance use disorder (SUD) patient records. 89 Fed. Reg. 12472, Feb. 16, 2024. https://www.govinfo.gov/content/pkg/FR-2024-02-16/pdf/2024-02544.pdf. Accessed 29 Apr 2024.

Chapter 3
Equity and Telemedicine

Crystal-Rose Cuellar

As the entire world changed and adjusted to the COVID-19 pandemic, so did our healthcare delivery systems. The rapid expansion of telemedicine services was vital in early stages of the pandemic. The expansion was dramatic and incredible. Between March 2019 and March 2020, there was a remarkable 4347% telehealth claim line increase nationally [1]. The mass transition to telemedicine aimed to reduce unnecessary virus exposure for the patients and providers, limit disruption to healthcare delivery (including acute, routine, primary, and specialty care), and improve access to care in the setting of a global shutdown. Public health emergency orders recognized the advantages of telehealth with protections in reimbursement, flexibility in virtual formats which were previously restricted under the Health Insurance Portability and Accountability Act (HIPAA), and modified out-of-state licensing requirements [2]. The benefits of telehealth were seemingly obvious for adolescent and adult patients alike. In fact, colloquially and professionally, telemedicine was considered a possible "virtually perfect solution." [3]

While telemedicine was a solution for many, it also became clear that the virtual format was potentially fraught with equity challenges and limitations. Racial and ethnic minorities were already facing disproportionate rates of COVID-19 [4]. This was compounded by the existing health disparities that have resulted from a long-standing history of structural racism and limited healthcare access. As such, these populations were among the highest need for care in the new virtual landscape. However, these were also the groups least likely to have access to the technology necessary for telemedicine and remained at risk for poorer health outcomes [5]. This example demonstrates that a clear understanding of the equity implications is necessary as we continue to optimize telemedicine in the post-COVID era of healthcare.

C.-R. Cuellar (✉)
Department of Pediatrics, University of Washington, Seattle, WA, USA
e-mail: Crystalrose.cuellar@seattlechildrens.org

Y. N. Evans et al. (eds.), *Telemedicine for Adolescent and Young Adult Health Care*, https://doi.org/10.1007/978-3-031-55760-6_3

The following case serves to demonstrate the limitations of telemedicine in terms of disparities and also highlight opportunities in equitable care.

Case

Xander is a 17-year-old assigned male at birth presenting to the school-based clinic for initial visit. He is a new student who has transferred from a rural town several hours away. He reports a history of "mild depression" and an eating disorder "that I don't really have anymore." He can't remember when his last well visit was or the name of his prior pediatrician. The nurse practitioner peruses the electronic medical record (EMR) for collateral information. Fortunately, outside records are accessible. She notices that he has very few visits over the past few years. The last in person visit was over 2 years ago. The EMR shows four telephone follow-ups regarding Xander's medication management for depression. There are several visits marked as "no show" thereafter with the medical provider as well as the clinic's dietitian and mental health therapist.

Xander recalls the telephone visits with some prompting. He remembers connecting to the last visit alone while babysitting his sibling while his parent was away at work. Xander reports that he did not refill his medication following the last telephone visit due to cost and transportation to the pharmacy. He also remembers that he was unable to attend subsequent video visits due to not having reliable Internet access or a smart device. The nurse practitioner proceeds to collect additional social history in the HEADSS exam: recent move was precipitated by housing instability after his parent was laid off from work; he is now living with extended family; he was previously in an online school program to allow time to help care for his younger siblings; and he reports worsening mental health after he lost touch with his friends. Objectively, his BMI has decreased from the 50th percentile to the 5th percentile since the last recorded value in his chart. His Patient Health Questionnaire-9 score is 15, suggesting "moderately severe depression."

Discussion

The example provided in the case demonstrates several factors that may contribute to inequitable access to telemedicine for adolescents. Access to appropriate technology is an important consideration. Inherently, telemedicine requires a patient to have appropriate Internet-enabled device with a viewable screen and video and audio capabilities. A patient also needs reliable access to Internet or cellular service to support the connection. These fundamental telemedicine requirements can lead to significant barriers in access to care.

Webber and colleagues surveyed patients in 2019 and 2020; they found that 30% of respondents had limited phone data, no data, or no phone. A higher proportion of patients with Medicaid had either a prepaid phone or no phone at all compared to patients with commercial insurance [6]. Curtis and colleagues detail similar findings of patients with no insurance or public insurance being significantly more likely to be without any digital access compared to those with private health insurance coverage [5]. The disparity was also apparent for racial/ethnic minority households: non-Hispanic Blacks, American Indian or Alaska natives, or Hispanics were more likely to be without any digital access compared to their non-Hispanic white counterparts. These findings are consistent with existing data demonstrating limited access to telemedicine technology for low-income households and racial/ethnic minorities [7, 8].

Further, as demonstrated in the case example, patients in rural households were found to be more likely to lack any digital access [5]. Even before the COVID-19 pandemic, health disparities existed for rural populations [9]. For adolescents, sub-specialty care (i.e., for specialized management of eating disorders, substance use, gender affirming care, etc.) is nearly non-existent in many rural regions [10]. Pre-COVID, telemedicine was thought to be an answer to bridging gaps in access to care for these remote populations. However, the rapidity of telemedicine expansion during the pandemic did not allow for the needed expansion in the broadband and technology access necessary for successful and equitable telemedicine implementation. It is estimated that a third of the rural population lacks the broadband access necessary for telemedicine services [11]. Without the means to access this healthcare service, the opportunity for equity barriers emerges.

The digital divide is also evident in the adolescent population specifically. Despite technological advances that have facilitated overall increases in access to Internet and technology, disparities have been persistent over time. In particular, Black and Hispanic adolescents continue to face disparities in Internet access and cell phone or smartphone use. The disparity is further exacerbated by socioeconomic status with significantly less low-income Black and Hispanic adolescents with access to the Internet or cell phones compared to high-income Black and Hispanic adolescents [12]. This is also consistent with more recent findings showing that children in low-income households or who are Black or Hispanic are less likely to have access to computers compared to higher income or white peers, respectively [13].

Black and Hispanic adolescents (in particular, those from low-income groups) were also more likely to use smartphone-only Internet (no home Internet access and no access via other devices) [11]. This may have important implications for telemedicine given that a smartphone connection needs to be strong enough to support a video visit and there may be a limit to Internet access based on data plans and specific videoconferencing phone applications compatible with telemedicine software.

Speaking a language other than English can represent additional factor leading to inequities. Since the COVID-19 pandemic, a number of studies have demonstrated less telemedicine utilization for non-English-speaking patients [14–16]. Although the adolescent patient themselves may speak English, having a family who speaks a language other than English may still relate to telemedicine inequities. For adolescents, many rely heavily on family to help navigate the healthcare system [17]. In regard to telehealth, this may include family coordinating with the clinic to schedule telemedicine appointment, receiving log-on instructions and links, troubleshooting technical setup or issues, and participating in the appointment. As such, language barriers may exist at any step in the telemedicine process that may lead to inequitable care delivery via telemedicine.

Evidence also supports the relationship between the above social determinants of health and inequities in both the primary care and specialty care sectors [18]. An important specialty to consider in the adolescent population is psychiatry and mental health. McBain and colleagues found that half of children and adolescents have inadequate access to psychiatric services in rural counties (compared to 3% in urban counties). Likewise mirroring the disparities previously discussed, children and adolescents in high-income counties had better access to psychiatric care (3% compared to 41% in low-income counties) [19]. Adolescents saw an increase in both psychiatric emergencies [20] as well as exacerbations in symptoms of OCD, eating disorders, PTSD, and other mental health diagnoses [21]. With an increase in healthcare needs but barriers in equitable access to the available telemedicine formats, disparities continued to grow for teenagers.

Despite the limitations and challenges in providing truly equitable care via telemedicine, the rapid transition to a virtual platform has had some positive impact and intent for vulnerable populations. First and foremost was the avoidance of unnecessary risks during the most critically contagious phase of the pandemic. With underserved populations at the highest risk of negative COVID-19 outcomes [4], the intent to protect patients served its purpose. Telemedicine also has the potential to address social determinants of health that contribute to health disparities. Telemedicine can improve access for those with transportation limitations. There is also a lower indirect cost for care by limiting the need for parental time off from work, travel, and childcare [22]. Patients generally report satisfaction with the virtual format and families whose lives are structured around work/childcare report appreciation of the convenience provided through telemedicine [23].

The telemedicine modality, whether videoconference or telephone, seems to make a difference for populations at highest risk for inequity. The technical requirements are more involved for videoconferencing and technical issues are more likely. Like the case presentation, telephone visits may be more accessible and some at risk groups may be more likely to have smartphone-only Internet access anyway [11]. Chang and colleagues showed that providers in high social vulnerability index areas were twice as likely to use phone as the primary telemedicine modality compared to those in low social vulnerability index areas [23]. This finding corroborates the notion that using the phone (without video) format may mitigate barriers to accessing care.

The advocacy for clinic and insurance reimbursement policies for audio-only (or telephone) visits may help bypass equity-related barriers to care. On a broader scale, efforts can continue to focus on maintaining reimbursement policies for telemedicine to ensure ready access to this format. Expanding broadband Internet access to rural communities has been an ongoing effort nationally. Providers should maintain a vigilant awareness of the potential threats to equity and intervene to mitigate the downstream effects of medical disparities. Device (tablet, hotspot, etc.) loaner programs, partnerships with community sites (libraries, schools, remote clinics, etc.), and avoidance of remote visits where appropriate are some strategies to consider [24]. Regardless, keeping equity a high priority is essential as our healthcare system moves into the post-COVID "new normal."

References

1. Gelburd R. Examining the state of telehealth during the COVID-19 pandemic. United Hospital Fund. https://uhfnyc.org/publications/publication/telehealth-during-covid-19. Published 29 June 2020.
2. https://telehealth.hhs.gov/providers/.
3. Hollander JE, Carr BG. Virtually perfect? Telemedicine for COVID-19. NEJM. 2020;382(18):1679–81.
4. Alcendor DJ. Racial disparities-associated COVID-19 mortality among minority populations in the US. J Clin Med. 2020;9(8):2442.
5. Curtis ME, Clingan SE, Guo H, Zhu Y, Mooney LJ, Hser YI. Disparities in digital access among American rural and urban households and implications for telemedicine-based services. J Rural Health. 2022;38(3):512–8.
6. Webber EC, McMillen BD, Willis DR. Health care disparities and access to video visits before and after the COVID-19 pandemic: findings from a patient survey in primary care. Telemed J E Health. 2022;28(5):712–9.
7. Lorence DP, Park H, Fox S. Racial disparities in health information access: resilience of the digital divide. J Med Sys. 2006;30(4):241–9.
8. Mitchell UA, Chebli PG, Ruggiero L, Muramatsu N. The digital divide in health-related technology use: the significance of race/ethnicity. Gerontol. 2019;59(1):6–14.
9. https://www.cdc.gov/ruralhealth/about.html.
10. Hahn SL, Burnette CB, Borton KA, Mitchell Carpenter L, Sonneville KR, Bailey B. Eating disorder risk in rural US adolescents: what do we know and where do we go? Int J Eat Disord. 2022;56(2):366–71.
11. https://www.fcc.gov/health/maps.
12. Dolcini MM, Canchola JA, Catania JA, Mayeda MMS, Dietz EL, Cotto-Negrón C, Narayanan V. National-level disparities in internet access among low-income and Black and Hispanic youth: Current population survey. J Med Internet Res. 2021;23(10):e27723.
13. Child Trends. Home computer access and internet use. https://www.childtrends.org/indicators/home-computer-access. Accessed 1 Feb 2021.
14. Linggonegoro DW, Sanchez-Flores X, Huang JT. How telemedicine may exacerbate disparities in patients with limited English proficiency. J Am Acad Dermatol. 2021;84(6):e289–90.
15. Qian AS, Schiaffino MK, Nalawade V, Aziz L, Pacheco FV, Nguyen B, et al. Disparities in telemedicine during COVID-19. Cancer Med. 2022;11(4):1192–201.
16. Xiong G, Greene NE, Lightsey HM IV, Crawford AM, Striano BM, Simpson AK, Schoenfeld AJ. Telemedicine use in orthopaedic surgery varies by race, ethnicity, primary language, and insurance status. Clin Orthop Relat Res. 2021;479(7):1417–25.
17. Lindstrom DP, Liu MM, Jira C. The role of parents and family networks in adolescent health-seeking in Ethiopia. JMF. 2019;81(4):830–46.
18. Eberly LA, Kallan MJ, Julien HM, Haynes N, Khatana SAM, Nathan AS, et al. Patient characteristics associated with telemedicine access for primary and specialty ambulatory care during the COVID-19 pandemic. JAMA Netw Open. 2020;3(12):–e2031640.

19. McBain RK, Cantor JH, Kofner A, Stein BD, Yu H. Ongoing disparities in digital and in-person access to child psychiatric services in the United States. JAACAP. 2022;61(7):926–33.
20. Choi KR, Martinez-Hollingsworth A, Mead M, Dappolonia MS. Adolescent psychiatric emergencies precipitated by the COVID-19 pandemic. J Psychosoc Nurs Ment Health Serv. 2021;59(7):17–21.
21. Palacio-Ortiz JD, Londoño-Herrera JP, Nanclares-Márquez A, Robledo-Rengifo P, Quintero-Cadavid CP. Psychiatric disorders in children and adolescents during the COVID-19 pandemic. Revista Colombiana de psiquiatria (English ed.). 2020;49(4):279–88.
22. Gurney J, Fraser L, Ikihele A, Manderson J, Scott N, Robson B. Telehealth as a tool for equity: pros, cons and recommendations. NZ Med J (Online). 2021;134(1530):111–5.
23. Chang JE, Lai AY, Gupta A, Nguyen AM, Berry CA, Shelley DR. Rapid transition to telehealth and the digital divide: implications for primary care access and equity in a post-COVID era. Milbank Q. 2021;99(2):340–68.
24. Ray KN, Keller D. Telehealth and pediatric care: policy to optimize access, outcomes, and equity. Pediatr Res. 2022;92:1496–9.

Chapter 4
Rural Populations

Julia Hadley, Sarah McHugh, Giselle Lambert, Cynthia Roleff, and Rachel Lescher

Introduction

Rural Communities and Health Disparities

Rural communities are defined by the US Census as any population, housing, and territory not included within an urbanized area (population > 50,000) or urban cluster (population 2500–50,000) [1]. Using this definition, 97% of the landmass of the United States is rural and home to approximately 20% of the population [2]. Many studies show those who live in rural areas have less access to healthcare and worse health outcomes compared to those who live in urban areas [3]. Adolescents in rural locations face similar disparities compared to adults and are less likely to be up to date on recommended vaccinations [4].

Though often categorized as a monolith, rural communities across the United States are diverse. Assessing needs only at a population level prevents providers from accurately identifying and effectively addressing health disparities. Research from the Centers for Disease Control and Prevention shows that Alaska Native/American Indian (AN/AI) people report poorer quality of life secondary to health-related conditions, increased rates of depression, and more frequent smoking use compared to non-Hispanic whites living in rural areas [3]. Similarly, survey respondents identifying as non-Hispanic Black, Hispanic, Asian, and Native Hawaiian/

J. Hadley · S. McHugh
Seattle Children's Hospital Pediatric Residency, University of Washington, Seattle, WA, USA

G. Lambert · C. Roleff
Alaska Native Tribal Health Consortium Telehealth Department, Anchorage, AK, USA
e-mail: gmlanbert@anthc.org; CJRoleff@anthc.org

R. Lescher (✉)
Alaska Native Medical Center Pediatric Endocrinology, Anchorage, AK, USA
e-mail: rlescher@southcentralfoundation.com

© The Author(s), under exclusive license to Springer Nature Switzerland AG 2024
Y. N. Evans et al. (eds.), *Telemedicine for Adolescent and Young Adult Health Care*, https://doi.org/10.1007/978-3-031-55760-6_4

Pacific Islander noted that cost was a barrier to healthcare and were less likely to have a primary care provider compared to non-Hispanic white survey respondents [3].

It is important to recognize both the overarching differences in providing healthcare in rural compared to urban settings and the specific disparities that may exist within an individual rural community. In this chapter, the Alaska Tribal Health System provides the framework for a discussion on effective expansion of healthcare delivery to adolescents in rural communities and the important role of telehealth in the delivery of high-quality care.

Description of Alaska and the Healthcare Framework

Alaska is the largest state geographically yet has the lowest population density in the nation. Alaska holds only 1.3 people per square mile [5] and a total population of approximately 733,000 people residing across 650,000 square miles [6]. Nearly half the population resides in one of Alaska's three largest cities: Anchorage, Fairbanks, and Juneau.

There are approximately 114,000 Alaska Native people living in Alaska, many of whom live in small villages [6]. Currently, there are 229 federally recognized tribes in the Alaska Region [7].

Access to Alaska Native villages can be difficult, with approximately 86% of municipalities in the state inaccessible by road [8]. Rural Alaska communities may also be embedded in protected lands or may be located in areas unsuitable for further road infrastructure, making expansion of access via motor vehicle impossible. Individuals in these areas often need to travel by plane for medical care, the costs of which are highly variable based on location, local resources, and urgency of travel based on illness severity.

The Alaska Native Tribal Health Consortium (ANTHC) does much to mitigate the disparities related to access. ANTHC is a nonprofit Tribal Health organization created to improve the health of all AN/AI individuals residing in Alaska. In partnership with the AN/AI people living in Alaska and the Tribal Health Organizations of the Alaska Tribal Health System, ANTHC oversees a coordinated and extensive network of healthcare throughout Alaska, using a "hub and spoke" model [9] (Fig. 4.1). The largest "hub" is the Alaska Native Medical Center, a tertiary care referral hospital in Anchorage that provides comprehensive medical services. The "spokes" are Regional Tribal Health Organization hospitals that provide primary and limited specialty care, along with their affiliated village clinics. Many of the village clinics are quite small and may be staffed by one or two community health workers who have undergone extensive healthcare training to provide primary care.

The ANTHC Telehealth department and Telehealth Technology Assessment Center serve as subject matter experts for the entire Alaska Tribal Health System. They provide guidance on telehealth hardware and software selection as well as the development of workflows. They also provide free trainings for Tribal partners.

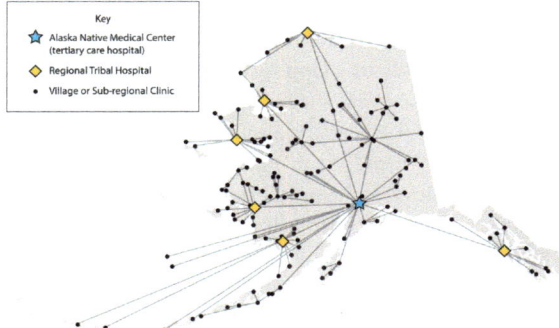

Fig. 4.1 Alaska Tribal Health System. The "hub and spoke" model: village and subregional clinics, identified by black dots; and connected by lines to the Regional Tribal Hospitals, identified by gold diamonds; and connected by lines to Alaska Native Medical Center, the tertiary care hospital in the Alaska Tribal Health System. (Image courtesy of the Alaska Native Tribal Health Consortium)

ANTHC and the other Tribal Health Organizations regularly collaborate on joint efforts, many of which are in the telehealth arena.

While the Alaska Tribal Health System strives to provide healthcare services close to families in remote areas, there is still a lack of access to advanced practitioners and physicians. Within the United States, 60% of the provider shortage is located in rural regions [10]. Telehealth is one modality that reduces the cost and increases accessibility to healthcare for those living in remote areas. A 2018 review by the American Academy of Pediatrics assessing telehealth usage found that for patients in remote areas, telehealth allows for improved triage and acute visits, reduced missed appointment rates, increased adherence to recommended therapies, and more appropriate frequency of recommended medical care visits [11]. Additionally, when appropriate, routine visits conducted via telehealth reduce the cost and burden of travel required for in-person visits from remote regions. These benefits all have the potential to promote health maintenance and improve disease management.

Telehealth is an important tool in delivering healthcare, but access to adequate broadband Internet and electronics to conduct such visits can be challenging in rural regions. The Telecommunications Act of 1996 and Federal Communications Commission (FCC) established a Rural Health Care Program with the goal of providing broadband internet to rural healthcare facilities [12]. However, according to data from 2018, 18.3 million Americans still lacked sufficient broadband access [12]. While 95% of Alaska households have a computer, only 87.3% have a broadband Internet subscription [6]. According to the FCC, Alaska villages have the least access to broadband Internet of all Alaska residents and all those occupying Tribal Lands throughout the United States [13]. In 2022, Alaska ranked as the worst state in the United States for low-priced broadband plans and the third worst state for broadband coverage [14]. Broadband Internet is extremely costly in rural Alaska. In some regions, the average monthly cost of home Internet can exceed $350 [15].

Multiple funded programs currently address broadband-related issues across the country, including the Telehealth Broadband Pilot. The Telehealth Broadband Pilot focuses on improving broadband mapping in select counties and boroughs across Alaska, Michigan, Texas, and West Virginia, with a goal of providing more accurate information to state and local efforts to deploy broadband infrastructure for healthcare and telehealth [16]. The program measures Internet speed through dedicated broadband measurement devices installed in clinics and homes, as well as through custom speed testing websites and smartphone applications available to the public in each state. The Telehealth Technology Assessment Center at ANTHC and the Rural Telehealth Evaluation Center at the University of Arkansas participate under this funding [16].

Cases: Rural Health and Telemedicine

As illustrated above, rural communities constitute unique populations who often have less access to care and poorer health outcomes compared to urban communities. Telehealth is one strategy employed to expand access to care. The following cases will highlight common challenges in providing care in rural areas. These areas include limited privacy in high occupancy houses and small communities, gaps in provider knowledge of local resources and difficulties when transferring patients to a higher level of care, and paucity of subspecialty services. The case discussions will seek to explore and provide solutions to these common problems.

Case 1: Rural Culture, Confidentiality and Privacy Concerns

A 17-year-old trans male presents for a telemedicine visit with his gender affirming care provider. Some of his family members are not aware of his gender identity. He lives in a small home with multiple people in a remote village and expressed he did not feel safe discussing concerns in front of his extended family. The patient's parents consented to the visit, and the patient then was able to go to a relative's home nearby to conduct the rest of the visit.

Adolescents across many communities and locations may feel uncomfortable discussing health issues in the presence of family members. The often tight-knit structure and culture of rural communities can present an additional barrier to privately discussing health concerns.

While each community is unique, rural community members often feel more important ties to location and have more positive civic sentiments, including placing higher value on family and community compared to their urban counterparts [17]. In small rural communities, it is common for teachers, physicians, religious leaders, law enforcement, or other authority figures to be well-known members of the community with multigenerational ties. This familiarity and intimate knowledge of the community can be beneficial when partnering with adolescents and understanding their experiences. Providers from the community may have more success building rapport and trust with an adolescent as they have a personal knowledge of the community and are not viewed as an outsider. However, this familiarity can also be a barrier to healthcare. When the local health provider is a family member or friend, adolescents may fear their personal health concerns or questions will not be kept confidential, or they may fear judgment from a respected or well-known person. Although rural communities are continually becoming more diverse with an influx of new inhabitants into these locations, [3] these areas may remain more homogenous than urban centers regarding political and social beliefs. It may be harder in these settings for individuals, particularly adolescents, to discuss aspects of their identity that may differ from the predominant views or norms within their community.

In addition to confidentiality concerns within small community social networks, the structure of homes in rural locations can make privacy during telehealth visits challenging. Households in rural communities are more likely to be multigenerational and experience overcrowding compared to those in urban environments [18]. In many rural regions, land is plentiful but high costs associated with transportation of material and labor in addition to high costs of fuel and rent can prevent development of more homes and result in overcrowding. According to the US Department of Housing and Urban Development, "overcrowded" is defined as more than 1 person per room, and "severely overcrowded" is defined as more than 1.5 people per room [18]. Throughout the United States, 2% of households are categorized as overcrowded with 1% categorized as severely overcrowded. Throughout Alaska, the rate is over twice as high for overcrowded and severely overcrowded households at 4% and 3% respectively, and in remote Alaska Native villages where cultures may support housing family members and others who have nowhere to stay, rates of overcrowding and severe overcrowding approach 50% of households [19]. The likelihood of having a private telehealth visit in one of these homes is very small.

Despite the added complexities of working in small communities with large household populations, confidentiality during a telehealth visit between a provider and the adolescent should be addressed similarly to an in-person visit. The provider can begin the telehealth visit by setting expectations and an agenda for the visit including a portion of the visit with all parties, followed by a private conversation between the provider and adolescent. Parents should be included in this initial conversation, whether it is prior to the appointment or as the appointment begins, to help establish trust between all party members. At the end of the visit, as is done for in-person visits, the provider should regroup with the adolescent and parent to summarize recommendations and arrange for follow-up.

During the confidential portion of the visit, providers should again remind teens of what can be kept confidential and what would need to be shared with others, including risk of harm to self or others or a laboratory result that may require public health notification, such as testing for sexually transmitted infections. The provider should then ensure that the adolescent feels that they are in an environment where they can talk in private and not be distracted. Finding a safe place to have a confidential discussion is not always easy.

The adolescent in the above case initially joined the visit from home and then transferred to a home with more privacy, both of which had adequate Internet connectivity. The home can be an ideal location, as it allows the provider to glean information and understand the adolescent's home environment and family dynamic. Depending on what a provider sees in a home, one may be able to identify psychosocial concerns that they might not have been privy to otherwise [12]. If the patient is unable to speak freely, the provider may suggest alternative ways of communicating to enhance privacy. This may include relocating to another room in the house, using headphones to keep provider to patient communication private, and/or messaging on a secure chat feature within the telehealth software if they feel uncomfortable speaking. Other alternatives can include having the provider ask binary questions while the adolescent wears headphones, using flashcards for yes/no, or using thumbs-up/down [12]. These methods are sub-optimal and should be used sparingly, as unconstrained verbal communication is the most fruitful and preferred.

If a private space within the home is not available, it may be feasible for the patient to leave the home. Depending on the time of year, weather, and network connection, it may be possible to have the adolescent or other members in the family step outside of the home for the appointment. In some northern cities in Alaska, temperatures during winter range from −10 to −55 degrees F, making speaking outside the home during winter months unlikely. Alternate locations could include a car outside the house or arranging time at the home of another friend or family member. It is important to discuss the plan for privacy in advance so that there are adequate accommodations.

Community centers or school-based clinics are useful locations to conduct telehealth visits, especially if a home visit is not secure, does not have reliable Internet, or otherwise compromises the integrity of the visit. Conducting telehealth visits at community clinics can be beneficial for the telehealth provider as the community health provider can obtain necessary vital sign measurements, do a physical exam as needed, and provide other resources when necessary. Privacy can then be provided within the clinic to complete any confidential discussions. The use of headsets, sound machines, and/or white noise generators in hallways can help further ensure privacy in small clinics.

School-based telehealth programs have also shown promising results for both acute and chronic care [20] and can provide a comfortable and secure location for adolescent telehealth appointments. These programs require a partnership between the schools and healthcare providers which often requires advance collaboration with legal departments, risk management, the school board, and others to ensure safe practices. Obtaining parental consent for a school visit may be the biggest challenge [21] but is a critical part of the visit. With school-based clinics, the teacher, school nurse, counselor, or another professional should designate a quiet area where the adolescent can conduct the visit and not be overheard or interrupted.

In many rural Alaska communities, local clinics and schools have more reliable Internet access than individual homes. If broadband Internet connectivity issues persist in these locations, video appointments may be converted to audio-only appointments if the adolescent and parent agree and if the provider feels a phone call will provide adequate information. While audio-only visits are an option, a generous portion of communication is lost, including facial expression and body language, and audio-only visits do not allow for visual physical examination.

If the adolescent still feels uncomfortable disclosing information due to their environment, or if the provider feels that there is significant hindrance to communication, the provider may need to end the visit. In these cases, it is best for the provider to work with the adolescent to find a different time or location in which to continue the conversation. The provider might find it helpful to obtain the adolescent's personal phone number or email to help set up a confidential visit time. The provider can also utilize mental health questionnaires via secure email or electronic health record to gather sensitive information from the adolescent prior to the next visit [22].

Key Takeaway Points

It is important for the provider to establish a framework for the visit including a confidential discussion for adolescent patients. For an adolescent patient in a rural community, finding privacy is often a complex task that requires brainstorming and problem solving. A community health clinic, school, home, and friend/relative's home are all possible options. Of utmost importance is that the adolescent feels they have a safe space to talk so that good rapport between provider and patient can be established and maintained.

Case 2: Utilization of Local Resources and Decision to Transfer Care

A 16-year-old with rheumatoid arthritis and depression presents for a routine follow-up visit with their rheumatologist via video telemedicine. The patient presents to their local clinic with the parent and community health worker present for the visit. The patient was tearful during the visit and agreed to have a private discussion with the physician. The physician discussed that confidentiality would be maintained during the private discussion unless the patient was imminently at risk of harm. During the confidential discussion, the patient disclosed worsening depression and anxiety, along with suicidal ideation. The patient had a plan for suicide, did not feel safe at home, and was worried about self-harm, disclosing that guns were accessible at the home. Although initially, the patient was reluctant to allow the physician to notify their parent, they eventually agreed and the physician spoke privately with the parent about the above concerns. The physician, parent, patient, and community health worker then rejoined to discuss next steps. Since there was no

*hospital at the remote site, the community health worker contacted an on-call pedi-
atrician in a regional hub to help urgently evacuate the patient first to the regional
hospital and subsequently to Anchorage for higher levels of care.*

In certain circumstances, especially under the guidance of community health
workers and local resources, telehealth may be used to avoid transfer to a higher
level of care by helping providers make assessments and triage patients [20]. This
can be valuable to the patient for several reasons. Travel is often particularly difficult for patients or their escorts who have disabilities. The cost of travel can also be
financially draining, and the time required to travel can take adolescents and their
escorts away from school and work for multiple days (e.g., it can take 3 days of
travel to get from some rural Alaska communities to the city of Anchorage). In a
person's own community, family, friends, and other trusted people familiar to their
needs and culture can provide support and resources, while patients who require
transfer out of their community are often separated from these cultural supports and
community strengths [23]. Travel to a larger city or regional hub can also be difficult
to navigate for people who live in small villages or towns and are not accustomed to
a large city with an international airport, busy multilane roads, and even elevators.
Nevertheless, there will be instances when the medical home may need to be
expanded. Telehealth allows for more equitable and just care for those living in
rural, remote communities by allowing the opportunity to access care and triage
more urgent healthcare needs.

Individuals living in rural communities across the United States have less access
to advanced practitioners or physicians than those in urban areas. Many rural places
lack the infrastructure to support a local clinic and those that do may have difficulty
recruiting advanced practitioners and physicians to work in these more isolated
locations. As a result, the use of community health workers (CHWs) has become
increasingly common. Though the role differs by state and community needs,
CHWs are often members of the community who undergo training to provide basic
medical care and navigation of health systems in locations without advanced practitioners or physicians. In the United States, there are over 125,000 CHW positions,
and the US Bureau of Labor Statistics predicts that these positions will increase by
more than 15% in the coming decade [24].

Within the Alaska Tribal Health System, Community Health Aides/Practitioners
(CHA/Ps) play a vital role in the care of patients in remote villages. CHA/Ps are
typically members of the local community with at least a high school degree who
undergo a series of health training and education. The program is managed by
ANTHC and supported by four training centers. Across the Alaska Tribal Health
System, there are four levels of CHA/Ps, each having completed a progressive combination of medical education and clinical practicum hours. The levels culminate in
a full Community Health Aid Practitioner. CHA/Ps learn basic skills in medical
interviewing, physical examination, and administration of medications. Currently,
there are approximately 550 certified CHA/Ps in more than 170 Alaska villages [9].
In many villages, CHA/Ps are the only medical staff routinely available to provide
immediate, hands-on healthcare for the community. Often the first point of entry
into the care system, CHA/Ps work closely with regionally based advanced

practitioners and physicians to evaluate and treat patients via electronic health record messages, phone calls, and video telemedicine.

CHA/Ps are often the subject matter experts regarding local community resources, customs, and languages. CHA/Ps can help to identify medical and mental health resources within the community that the patient and family can access. If resources are adequate, the telehealth provider can engage in shared decision-making with the adolescent, parent or guardian, and CHA/P. If the patient is not acutely ill, and all parties feel comfortable keeping the adolescent within their community, then it is often beneficial to do so. As appropriate, the telehealth provider can also refer the patient to the subregional clinic or regional hospital, which will still be closer to the patient's home than traveling to Anchorage.

When the medical home must be expanded, it is useful to understand the healthcare landscape. For instance, in the Alaska Tribal Health System, there are four levels of facility to which a patient's care may be escalated. Village clinics, primarily staffed by CHA/Ps, are the first medical contact for most rural patients. Small village clinics have limited resources. CHA/Ps can administer basic medications from a limited formulary, perform a small number of point-of-care tests (such as blood glucose and hemoglobin), and draw blood to be sent to the regional center. At subregional clinics, CHA/Ps can provide a higher level of care, depending on their scope of practice (level of training) and resources at each site. There are 25 of these centers throughout Alaska, and they are often equipped with a broader medication formulary, more substantial laboratory capabilities, and X-ray facilities. More in-person support is available at these facilities from rotating physician assistants, nurse practitioners, or physicians. For patients who require more extensive workup or inpatient hospitalization, the next escalation in care is to a regional hospital. In Alaska, the six tribal regional hospitals are staffed by physicians, nurse practitioners, and physician assistants and offer emergency departments serving as Level 4 trauma centers, inpatient services, and limited obstetric and other surgical interventions. If the regional hospital is not able to meet a patient's needs or additional specialty services are required, the patient is usually transferred to Alaska Native Medical Center in Anchorage, the secondary and tertiary care referral center for the Alaska Tribal Health System.

As previously discussed, many rural communities are not on road systems. Even for those that are, the immediate need for transfer to a higher level of care may require air transportation. The adolescent in the above case required transfer of care from a remote village to the regional hospital and ultimately to the tertiary referral center, a trip requiring multiple expensive flights. To get from a rural village to a regional hospital, the patient usually will fly in a small aircraft (many times as small as a propeller plane which seats four or five people). From the regional hospital to the referral center, the patient would take a small commercial jet. According to current fares, average costs for a flight from a village to a regional center for two people (a minor plus an escort) are about $500 each, and from a regional center to Anchorage, it is approximately $700 each. For patients requiring urgent medical evacuation, the cost can be upward of $30,000 per flight [25]. In addition, from the initial point of care, many patients have to use alternative means to get to the nearest landing strip. Families may take snow machines (also called snowmobiles), four-wheelers, or dog teams across wild land to seek care at clinics from nearby villages. During winter months, families living near a river may use the frozen river as an ice road, driving their vehicles or snow machines to the clinic or regional hospital. In the summer, these families may use boats to travel along the river. From there, they can take the remaining flight(s) as necessary.

When the medical team determines that a patient needs a higher level of care, the acuity of illness and urgency of transfer are important decisions they must make. Commercial flights, even for serious medical issues, may take hours or days to arrange due to availability of pilots and flying conditions. For an adolescent in crisis, ground transportation or commercial flights may still be appropriate if they are able to be under the constant supervision of a caregiver. If the medical team determines that the patient needs urgent or emergent transfer (e.g., due to concern for ingestion, imminent self-harm, or injuries that need immediate attention), then the adolescent should have a medical evacuation flight arranged. At times, weather or limited flights delay even medical evacuation flights. In these cases, the telehealth provider can partner with the CHA/P and other providers as well as with the patient and their caregivers to establish a safe contingency plan until the adolescent can access the healthcare they need.

Key Takeaway Points

This case highlights an acute issue requiring transfer for more intensive therapy and how effective communication among the patient, family, local and regional health providers, and the telehealth provider improved care for this adolescent. Without telehealth, this patient would not have had the opportunity to disclose their concerns to the provider and get the care they ultimately needed. In this case, the risks associated with travel outweighed the benefits of having the adolescent stay within their community, and the use of telehealth acted as an adjunct for diagnosis, discussion, and determination of final disposition. With other cases that do not require escalated levels of care, the use of telehealth and triaging abilities enables providers to strive to keep patients in their home communities whenever safely possible.

Case 3: Subspecialty Services and Maintaining Standards of Care

A 15-year-old with type I diabetes presents for routine subspecialty endocrinology follow-up via *telemedicine. She lives in a remote village that has a community health aide, and the closest physician to her is a family medicine physician who is at least 50 miles away. Every 3 months, she needs follow-up for her diabetes, including vital signs, a detailed physical exam, reviewing home glucose and medication records, and laboratory monitoring. Without reliable home Internet, she goes to the local community clinic to connect with her subspecialty provider* via *video telemedicine.*

Maintaining Standards of Care

Diabetes management is a useful example for extrapolation to other conditions when considering the utility of telemedicine in chronic disease [26]. Pediatric diabetes management requires consideration of various challenges such as family dynamics, school support, progression through developmental stages, physiologic changes with growth and puberty, and advances in diabetes technology. Given these and other factors, adolescents and their families are best served by working with a multidisciplinary team including the primary care provider, diabetes specialist, diabetes educator, dietitian, and mental health professional. Regular visits with the team are necessary to improve education and support for diabetes self-management, nutrition therapy, and psychosocial support, as well as for monitoring for and treating complications and related conditions [27].

Emerging studies show that in rural populations, telemedicine is safe and effective at improving glycemic control [28]. During telemedicine diabetes visits, patients and their families can meet with the diabetes specialist, diabetes educator, dietitian, and mental health professional. Home glucose monitoring and insulin use data can be shared using secure cloud-based technology. Laboratory monitoring to screen for related conditions can be performed at the patient's primary medical home. The use of remote monitoring tools such as real-time continuous glucose monitoring can also allow the diabetes team to intervene sooner if problems arise and allow patients and their families to communicate more effectively with the provider. During telehealth visits, the local provider can be more involved in the care by participating in the visit as needed, downloading and reviewing glucose logs, performing laboratory testing, reviewing and transmitting imaging, and refilling medications and supplies.

The Need for Rural Subspecialty Services

Children have high rates of chronic disease requiring complex management, with an estimated 19% needing specialty care [29]. Approximately 25% of children who need complex management have difficulty obtaining subspecialty care [29]. The availability of pediatric subspecialists is even lower than that of adult subspecialists, as children historically have fewer chronic subspecialty disease management needs when compared to adults [30].

Most pediatric subspecialists are located in urban centers, making access to subspecialty care even harder for children in rural communities. An estimated one in three pediatric patients requiring subspecialty care must travel more than 40 miles to see a subspecialist [31]. The length of travel increases significantly for those in more geographically remote areas. The ability to access pediatric subspecialty care also becomes increasingly difficult with the distance a patient lives from a referral center and the degree of poverty in a community [30]. This indicates that geographic barriers can further exacerbate already present health inequities in vulnerable populations. Telemedicine can help decrease these barriers by making access to subspecialty care more widely available.

As with diabetes, complex management of chronic pediatric diseases often requires frequent laboratory and/or radiographic monitoring, physical exams, and follow-up appointments. For families living in remote regions, this can create a large financial and time burden. Families coming from rural areas may spend multiple days traveling to an appointment, require lodging at their destination, and miss multiple days of work and school. The use of telehealth can help mitigate some of these barriers to care while also providing quality care for patients and families [20].

A 2017 study by Brophy found that monitoring children with end-stage renal disease monthly via telehealth in conjunction with quarterly in-person visits saved families more than $500 in travel, lodging, and meals over a 1-year time span [32]. For most rural Alaskans, the cost savings are much greater. Similarly, a 2016 study by Dayal et al. found that rates of emergency department utilization and hospital admission for patients with neurologic disorders were four times lower in patients who received telehealth in their local community compared with patients who traveled to in-person appointments [33]. These studies suggest that improving access to subspecialty care using telehealth prevents unnecessary medical care, reduces costs to families, and limits daily disruptions at school and work.

While telehealth has many benefits for direct patient care, it can also be a useful tool for education, consultation, and support of local medical providers in rural locations. Rural providers often provide the initial management of children and adolescents requiring subspecialty care as they confront delays in access to subspecialty centers due to financial, physical, or geographic barriers. Project ECHO (Extension for Community Healthcare Outcomes) is a "hub and spoke" model of telehealth that connects groups of subspecialty providers from academic centers with rural community clinicians. In these telehealth sessions, subspecialists can provide case-based teachings and general knowledge to community healthcare providers to help increase the quality of care for complex patients in rural locations [10]. Rural providers also have the opportunity to submit cases for discussion with the whole team. There are also many less formalized systems of connecting subspecialists with primary care pediatricians such as subspecialty hotline services which can help with acute management and stabilization, long-term care plans, and assistance with referrals. Rural providers have found these services to be particularly helpful in management and stabilization when inclement weather delays transfer of acutely ill patients as well as for initiation of treatment for subacute illnesses while patients await subspecialty appointments [34].

Subspecialists benefit from telehealth in a number of ways as well. When treating patients with chronic diseases, the relationship formed between a patient and their specialist can improve the health and well-being of the patient. With the removal of barriers of travel, time away from school and work, and cost, the use of telehealth can contribute to reduced missed appointments and sufficient frequency of visits [11]. By increasing use of telehealth, the subspecialist can meet the patient's local healthcare team and collaborate for the patient's health needs while removing barriers of travel, time away from school and work, and cost. They can learn about the resources and barriers to care in their patients' communities. In-home telehealth visits allow the provider to meet other family members who may not be able to accompany the patient to their specialty visits but who also help care for the patient at home. In-school telehealth visits allow the subspecialty provider to work directly with the teachers, aides, and nurses who help care for the adolescent during the school day. This expands the patient's medical home, thereby improving overall care.

In addition to telehealth, the use of field health clinics is another way to augment adolescent subspecialty care. Field health clinics are common practice in Alaska, with the subspecialist traveling to a regional site quarterly. This helps to reduce travel burden for the patients, though they still must travel from the village to the regional site. The field health clinic also provides benefit to the subspecialist by allowing the visiting provider to learn more about the needs and resources in that region, foster relationships with the regional care providers, and see patients in person without as significant cost and time of travel falling to patients and their families. Many patients with chronic diseases have disabilities that make travel more difficult, making field health clinics and telehealth optimal alternatives.

Key Takeaway Points

Telehealth can be an effective tool in expanding subspecialty services both in the form of direct patient care and partnership and continuing educational opportunities with rural providers. Telehealth appointments can reduce the cost, travel, and time burden placed on rural patients who require frequent medical care. The use of community health aides or community health workers can serve as important extensions of the subspecialty provider to assist with patient education, medication management, physical examinations, and collection of labs to maintain the standard of care for patients with chronic or complex illnesses.

Summary

Adolescents in rural communities confront many barriers to medical care, many of which may be improved by access to telehealth. The three cases above highlight some of the specific challenges that rural adolescents may encounter including challenges with confidentiality in small communities, access to higher levels of care and emergency services, and accessibility of subspecialty services. Though reliable and affordable Internet access can be an additional challenge in rural communities, telehealth is still a compelling and effective tool in overcoming barriers in order to provide patients with the same standard of care as their urban counterparts. Knowledge of local resources, including community clinics and health care providers, can help to further expand the use of telehealth for both direct patient care as well as rural provider consultation and education.

References

1. United States Census Bureau. Urban and Rural. 2022. https://www.census.gov/programs-surveys/geography/guidance/geo-areas/urban-rural.html. Accessed 28 Apr 2022.
2. Ratcliffe M, Burd C, Holder K, Fields A. Defining rural at the U.S. Census Bureau 2022. https://www.census.gov/library/publications/2016/acs/acsgeo-1.html. Accessed 19 Apr 2022.
3. James CV, Moonesinghe R, Wilson-Frederick SM, Hall JE, Penman-Aguilar A, Bouye K. Racial/ethnic health disparities among rural adults—United States, 2012–2015. MMWR Surveill Summ. 2017;66:1–9. https://doi.org/10.15585/mmwr.ss6623a1.
4. Tsai Y, Lindley MC, Zhou F, Stokley S. Urban-rural disparities in vaccination service use among low-income adolescents. J Adolesc Health. 2021;69:114–20.
5. Allhoff F, Golemon L. Rural bioethics: the Alaska context. HEC Forum. 2020;32:313–31.
6. United States Census Bureau. Census Bureau QuickFacts: Alaska. 2022. https://www.census.gov/quickfacts/fact/table/AK/PST045221. Accessed 26 Apr 2022.
7. Dhss.alaska.gov. Alaska Primary Care Needs Assessment. 2016. https://dhss.alaska.gov/dph/Emergency/Documents/healthcare/Primary%20Care%20Needs%20Assessment/AlaskaPrimaryCareNeedsAssessment_2015_2016.pdf. Accessed 26 Apr 2022.
8. Labor.alaska.gov. 2017 Population estimates by borough, census area, and economic region 2017. http://www.labor.alaska.gov/news/2019/news19-01_data.pdf. Accessed 26 Apr 2022.
9. CHAP Alaska. Community health aide program—CHAP Alaska. 2022. https://akchap.org/community-health-aide/. Accessed 19 Apr 2022.
10. Marcin JP, Shaikh U, Steinhorn RH. Addressing health disparities in rural communities using telehealth. Pediatr Res. 2015;79:169–76.
11. Olson CA, McSwain SD, Curfman AL, Chuo J. The current pediatric telehealth landscape. Pediatrics. 2018;141:e2017234.
12. Curfman A, McSwain SD, Chuo J, Yeager-McSwain B, Schinasi DA, Marcin J, Herendeen N, Chung SL, Rheuban K, Olson CA. Pediatric telehealth in the COVID-19 pandemic era and beyond. Pediatrics. 2021;148:e2020047795.
13. Federal Communications Commission. 2020 Broadband Deployment Report 2020. https://www.fcc.gov/reports-research/reports/broadband-progress-reports/2020-broadband-deployment-report. Accessed 10 Apr 2022.
14. Cooper T, Tanberk J. Best and worst states for internet coverage, prices and speeds, 2021—Broadband Now. 2022. https://broadbandnow.com/research/best-states-with-internet-coverage-and-speed. Accessed 20 Apr 2022.
15. Alaska Public Media. With $350 monthly internet bills, Y-K Delta residents face high hurdle for connectivity. Alaska Public Media; 2022. https://www.alaskapublic.org/2021/03/04/with-350-monthly-internet-bills-y-k-delta-residents-face-high-hurdle-for-connectivity/. Accessed 19 Apr 2022
16. Office for the Advancement of Telehealth. 2021. In: Official web site of the U.S. Health Resources & Services Administration. https://www.hrsa.gov/rural-health/telehealth. Accessed 2 May 2022.
17. Ulrich-Schad JD, Duncan CM. People and places left behind: work, culture and politics in the rural United States. J Peasant Stud. 2018;45:59–79.

18. United States Census Bureau. Measuring Overcrowding in Housing. 2007. https://www.census.gov/programs-surveys/ahs/research/publications/Measuring_Overcrowding_in_Hsg.html Accessed 2 May 2022.
19. Wiltse N, Madden D. Cold Climate Housing Research Center for Alaska Housing Finance Corporation. 2018 Alaska housing assessment: statewide housing summary. https://www.ahfc.us/application/files/3115/1638/5454/2018_Statewide_Housing_Assessment_-_Part_1_-_Executive_Summary_and_Housing_Needs_011718.pdf. Accessed 2 May 2022.
20. Curfman AL, Hackell JM, Herendeen NE, Alexander JJ, Marcin JP, Moskowitz WB, Bodnar CEF, Simon HK, SD MS, AAP Section on Telehealth Care, Committee on Practice and Abmulatory Medicine, Committee on Pediatric Workforce. Telehealth: opportunities to improve access, quality, and cost in pediatric care. Pediatrics. 2022;149:e2021056035.
21. Burke BL Jr, Hall RW, Section on Telehealth Care. Telemedicine: pediatric applications. Pediatrics. 2015;136:e293–308.
22. Evans YN, Golub S, Sequeira GM, Eisenstein E, North S. Using telemedicine to reach adolescents during the COVID-19 pandemic. J Adolesc Health. 2020;67:469–71.
23. Pignatiello A, Teshima J, Boydell KM, Minden D, Volpe T, Braunberger PG. Child and youth telepsychiatry in rural and remote primary care. Child Adolesc Psychiatric Clin N Am. 2011;20:13–28.
24. Washburn DJ, Callaghan T, Schmit C, Thompson E, Martinez D, Lafleur M. Community health worker roles and their evolving interprofessional relationships in the United States. J Interprof Care. 2021;545:1–7.
25. Air Ambulance Services in the United States. FAIR Health. 2021. https://s3.amazonaws.com/media2.fairhealth.org/whitepaper/asset/Air%20Ambulance%20Services%20in%20the%20United%20States%20-%20A%20Study%20of%20Private%20and%20Medicare%20Claims%20-%20A%20FAIR%20Health%20White%20Paper.pdf. Accessed 2 May 2022.
26. Wang H, Yuan X, Wang J, Sun C, Wang G. Telemedicine maybe an effective solution for management of chronic disease during the COVID-19 epidemic. Prim Health Care Res Dev. 2021;22:e48. https://doi.org/10.1017/S1463423621000517.
27. American Diabetes Association Professional Practice Committee. 14. Children and adolescents: standards of medical care in diabetes–2022. Diabetes Care. 2022;45(Suppl 1):S208–31.
28. American Diabetes Association Professional Practice Committee. 1. Improving care and promoting health populations: standards of medical care in diabetes–2022. Diabetes Care. 2022;45(Suppl 1):S8–S16.
29. Bethell CD, Kogan MD, Strickland BB, Schor EL, Robertson J, Newacheck PW. A national and state profile of leading health problems and health care quality for US children: key insurance disparities and across-state variations. Acad Pediatr. 2011;11(3 Suppl):S22–33.
30. Mayer ML. Disparities in geographic access to pediatric subspecialty care. Maternal Child Health J. 2008;12:624–32.
31. Mayer ML. Are we there yet? Distance to care and relative supply among pediatric medical subspecialties. Pediatrics. 2006;118:2313–21.
32. Brophy PD. Overview on the challenges and benefits of using telehealth tools in a pediatric population. Adv Chronic Kidney Dis. 2017;24:17–21.
33. Dayal P, Chang CH, Benko WS, Pollock BH, Crossen SS, Kissee J, Ulmer AM, Hoch JS, Warner L, Marcin JP. Hospital utilization among rural children served by pediatric neurology telemedicine clinics. JAMA Netw Open. 2019;2:e199364.
34. Ray KN, Demirci JR, Bogen DL, Mehrotra A, Miller E. Optimizing telehealth strategies for subspecialty care: recommendations from rural pediatricians. Telemed J E Health. 2015;21:622–9.

Chapter 5
Telehealth and Medical Education

Sarah A. Golub

Introduction

The explosion of telemedicine with the onset of COVID-19 made the impossible feat of continuing clinical care during a global pandemic a reality. In the early phases of the pandemic, Adolescent medicine providers described the benefits and challenges of reaching youth through virtual clinical encounters; to our relief, young people not only seemed amenable to receiving virtual care but were facile in adopting the technology necessary to conduct these encounters [1]. True to the interdisciplinary and collaborative nature of those working in the field, leaders in adolescent health came together to share early lessons learned in times of change and the impact on academic programming in adolescent medicine divisions throughout the country [2]. A common thread among academicians and medical providers across all specialties however was the challenge of how to support medical trainees during this time of unprecedented chaos. Underprepared for the rapid transition to telehealth, medical educators were left to improvise on how to incorporate learners into this new form of care delivery. While in the early months efforts were made to keep "nonessential" team members at home to prevent infection transmission and minimize use of personal protective equipment (PPE), the compelling voices of trainees as well as health educators were heard, emphasizing the importance of keeping learners involved in care for several key reasons: to improve patient health, to extend the capabilities of health care teams and systems, to provide experiential learning, and to increase student and trainees' professional identity formation in ensuring they become competent, caring and empathic physicians [3, 4].

S. A. Golub (✉)
Division of Adolescent Medicine, Seattle Children's Hospital, University of Washington School of Medicine, Seattle, WA, USA
e-mail: Sarah.golub@seattlechildrens.org

© The Author(s), under exclusive license to Springer Nature
Switzerland AG 2024
Y. N. Evans et al. (eds.), *Telemedicine for Adolescent and Young Adult Health Care*, https://doi.org/10.1007/978-3-031-55760-6_5

Integration of medical learners into telehealth has come as a challenge to many of us still struggling to master this method of clinical care delivery ourselves. However, many of the medical students and trainees of today have grown up in an era where they have been surrounded by digital technology and are often more comfortable than supervising faculty with communicating and processing information by means of virtual or electronic modalities. This generation of "digital natives," while technologically savvy, still needs and deserves formalized training to develop their skills in delivering high-quality care via telemedicine [5, 6]. Medical educators have called for the cultivation of "webside manner," to complement "bedside manner," as a separate skillset to be included in medical training [7]. Prior to the pandemic, telemedicine training for medical students, residents, and even clinical faculty was minimal, and educators had limited skills on how to effectively teach learners through this modality [8]. This has slowly begun to shift since March 2020 with the COVID-19 pandemic cultivating the development of new teaching strategies, adaptation of "tele-teaching" to facilitate remote education, and trainees readily adjusting to a new learning environment [9, 10]. As such, despite the many horrors of the pandemic, some "silver linings" can be found in the acceleration of positive change in the advancement of health care education [11].

Approaches to Telehealth Workflow with Learners

Regardless of their discipline, medical educators, by virtue of their training, have been exposed to countless styles and techniques in clinical teaching, and many have finessed and honed these skills over time. The current literature in the medical education realm offers evidence-based models providing guidance around bedside teaching [12]. With the rapid transition to virtual care however, medical educators were unprepared to teach learners and were left to draw on their own creativity to explore effective strategies to incorporate students and trainees at all levels into the care they were providing.

Virtual telehealth consults, both in the inpatient and outpatient settings, have been described as successful collaborative experiences between attending physicians and trainees in various specialties including surgery, otolaryngology, dermatology, allergy, and rheumatology [13–17]. Several modes of clinical precepting have been utilized in telehealth encounters. In most published models, the learner first logs into the virtual platform, interacts with the patient, obtains relevant medical history, and leaves the virtual room (or temporarily returns the patient to the virtual "waiting room") to present the patient to the attending. After discussion, both the learner and the attending re-enter the virtual space (or bring patient out of the "waiting room") to complete the visit with the patient/family [13]. Others have advocated for a model of virtual "triangle teaching," when the patient remains present during the discussion between the learner and preceptor, and the learner presents using patient-accessible language free of medical jargon [18, 19]. This method has been utilized prior to the transition to virtual clinical care and is similar to the practice of "family-centered rounds" which has historically been used in the inpa-tient setting [20]. Recent evidence suggests that patients have been receptive to this modality in telemedicine visits [15].

An alternate variation on telehealth clinic flow is having the learner lead a tele-health visit while the preceptor is present in the virtual room with audio and video capabilities disabled. This allows for enhanced autonomy for the learner and per-haps a more relaxed feel of the visit for the patient, without the overt presence of an audience. This modality has been found to be valued by learners for two reasons. The first is the ability of the learner to be directly observed by the attending and thus have the opportunity to receive direct feedback on their interviewing skills and com-munication techniques, both crucial competencies particularly as they pertain to adolescent care. The second is that it allows for the preceptor to send the learner a direct text message during the interview, either through the virtual platform or a separate HIPPA-compliant platform, to assist the learner with any in-the-moment prompts during the encounter. In one study, trainees in an adolescent medicine rota-tion reported highly valuing this method, describing it as a unique learning oppor-tunity that would not be as accessible in a traditional clinical precepting model [21].

In addition to the above examples, there may be scenarios involving sensitive topics or patient preference for discretion, when the attending physician prefers to lead the visit independently. With permission from the patient however, the attend-ing may choose to invite the learner(s) to observe the encounter with their audio and video disabled. To distinguish this from passive "shadowing," medical educators have suggested means to keep the learner actively engaged through this model by inviting them to listen for specific components of the interview and be prepared for discussion after the visit (e.g., "Listen to the language I use while obtaining a sexual history") [18].

Clinical Teaching Strategies for Telehealth

While the clinical workflow paradigms above have been described in the literature, to date, few studies have formally analyzed the effectiveness of various teaching strategies with telehealth. Several techniques however have been described and pro-moted to support educators in virtual clinical precepting since the onset of the COVID-19 pandemic (see Table 5.1) [22].

Pre-Huddle with Learner

Advanced preparation for a telemedicine visit with a learner is important in devel-oping a plan for the clinic session. This is an opportunity to determine which patients will be seen and establish the leaner's role for each visit if appropriate. The use of an electronic huddle (e-huddle) used by some institutions and sent to the learner at

Table 5.1 Best practices for conducting telehealth encounters with trainees [22]

Pre-visit	During visit	Post-visit
Pre-huddle with learner Identify learning goals Review clinical case Anticipate technology failures Prepare learner to receive feedback	Actively include learner in the visit Invite learner to ask questions Provide learner with autonomy when appropriate Observe learners' interview skills and style	Debrief case Review relevant clinical pearls or literature Invite learner's self-reflection of their role in visit Provide feedback

least 1 day prior to clinic has been reported by trainees as an effective strategy to help facilitate clear communication [23]; this can also be used as a means to prompt trainees to review select patient charts as indicated by their preceptor. Other preceptors may choose to pre-huddle by telephone or by logging onto the telehealth video conference platform just prior to the start of the first visit. The huddle also allows a preceptor to review relevant literature or resources to help prepare the learner to be knowledgeable in leading a visit. Attending physicians may also choose to use this time to review expectations around clinical documentation. Team huddles have been found to be effective in modeling interdisciplinary and collaborative care for learners in other hospital settings [24].

Identify Learning Objectives of Trainee

As part of a pre-clinic discussion, it is beneficial to cultivate a relationship with the learner and to understand their learning goals for the session. Though this can pose more of a challenge in a virtual setting than in person, preceptors should be intentional about ascertaining a learner's clinical interests and any particular skills they hope to hone during the clinic. Tailoring the educational experience to the individual creates a more positive and welcoming learning environment for the student or trainee. Preceptors may also notify learner that they will offer real-time feedback after each telehealth visit which can be targeted to their specific learning goals.

Anticipate Possible Technology Challenges

Prior to initiating a telehealth encounter, learners should be encouraged to practice with the selected telehealth platform if it is not yet familiar to them. The learner and preceptor should develop a plan for an alternative communication mechanism should their telehealth connection with the patient fail at any point during the visit. This might include switching to a mobile hotspot or alternative Internet connection if accessible, disabling video function to optimize Internet speed in low bandwidth environments, or switching to a telephone call. As such, it may be advantageous for the learner and preceptor to exchange phone numbers to allow for efficient communication should this occur. Secure text messages can also offer another solution for rapid communication if other technology modalities fail [22].

Engage Learner in Telemedicine Visit

If the attending physician is leading a visit, active learner observation and participation should be encouraged. As it is difficult to read nonverbal cues, clinical teachers can intentionally invite learners to ask questions or perform parts of the virtual visit such as obtaining a confidential social history from a patient if appropriate. Learners should also be encouraged to take notes when questions arise, which can be discussed at the conclusion of the visit. If the learner is leading the visit, preceptors can consider giving the learner autonomy by either being absent from the virtual room for the initial portion of the visit or disabling their audio and video functions.

Debrief Visit, Provide, and Elicit Feedback

With the loss of "hallway teaching," or time spent with learners between in-person appointments, it is important for preceptor and learner to remain on the virtual platform after the patient has left the room or reconnect shortly after by phone to debrief about the visit. This is an opportunity to review post-visit orders and plan, answer any clinical questions from the trainee relevant to the visit, or discuss any unique, complex, or challenging aspects of the encounter. If the attending has observed all or parts of the clinical encounter, invite the learner to self-reflect on the components they led. For instance, were there aspects of the interview they might phrase differently next time? Finally, provide direct feedback to the learner with a focus on their telehealth communication skills.

Cases: Scenarios of Telehealth Encounters with Learners

Case 1

A pediatric resident is working with you in your telemedicine clinic this afternoon. You have sent an e-huddle to the resident the day prior to clinic, indicating you would like them to lead the visit for a 17-year-old cisgender female (she/her pronouns) who is scheduled to see you for follow-up regarding painful menses. You have arranged for the resident to meet you in your Zoom virtual room 10 minutes before the clinic session begins for a pre-huddle, and you log on. You begin by asking the resident about their anticipated career plans and inquire about their experience thus far in residency with outpatient adolescent health, their comfort with telehealth, and any specific skills they would like to work on during today's clinic. The resident explains that they plan to work in pediatric primary care upon graduation, and they would like to improve their knowledge and understanding of contraception management. You take a moment to email the resident a helpful patient handout on contraceptive methods and briefly discuss the contraindications to estrogen-containing methods, including migraine with aura, which this patient has. After your pre-huddle, the medical assistant rooms the patient and alerts you that she is ready for her visit. You and the resident enter the virtual platform with the patient. You both introduce yourselves, and you ask the patient if she would be comfortable allowing the resident to lead the visit. She agrees, and you proceed to turn off your video and observe the resident during the encounter. You watch as they gather interim history. As the visit draws to a close, you send the resident a message with the chat function reminding them to ask if the patient has been using any barrier methods for prevention of pregnancy/STIs. The resident notes your message and asks the patient. As the conversation progresses and the patient expresses interest in contraception, you observe as the resident screenshares the contraception handout and listen as they outline options for the patient, who has decided she would prefer a levonorgestrel IUD. When the resident has completed this phase of the visit, they place the patient back in the virtual waiting room and you enable your video again and listen as the resident briefly reviews their assessment and plan. You agree that the resident has thoroughly reviewed options and that an IUD would be an excellent choice for diminishing bleeding and cramping for this patient. She is invited back into the virtual clinic room, where you reiterate that you agree with the plan and support the patient's choice, and you share details on bleeding patterns to anticipate with an IUD and provide an overview of the insertion process. You provide the next steps for her to schedule a LARC insertion in clinic with you the following week. After the patient has left the virtual platform, you debrief with the resident. They reflect that next time they might word some of their social history questions differently and will remember to ask about barrier methods. They report feeling more confident in understanding which methods contain estrogen vs progestin-only methods. You applaud them for building easy rapport with the patient and for validating her concerns about the IUD insertion procedure. You both log off the virtual platform to allow the resident to complete their note prior to starting the next telehealth visit.

Key Takeaway Points

A pre-huddle is an excellent opportunity to prepare a learner for any clinical pearls that will be useful during a clinical encounter. The ability to directly observe a trainee and provide real-time feedback can be extremely beneficial to learners.

Case 2

A 4th-year medical student is scheduled to be working with you in your virtual eating disorder clinic today. You will be seeing a 13-year-old nonbinary youth (they/them pronouns) with depression, recent history of hospitalization for suicidality, and restrictive eating who is new to your clinic. The day prior to clinic, you sent the student an e-huddle including an article on the diagnostic criteria for anorexia nervosa. You meet the student on Zoom for your planned pre-huddle before clinic. You learn that the student has had no experience caring for patients with eating disorders, but they did review the article you had sent. Given the sensitive nature of the visit due to recent SI, you plan for the student to be an active observer of the telehealth visit. Prior to the visit, you ask them to listen carefully for the language you use particularly in asking about disordered eating behaviors, body image, mood, and safety. You begin the visit together and ask for the patient/family's permission for the student to observe the visit. They agree, and the student disables their audio and video function. During the confidential portion of the visit, the patient discloses ongoing thoughts of self-harm in the setting of a recent trauma. The medical student listens as you model empathic listening and as you assess for imminent safety risk. You have a social worker follow up with the family to provide additional resources regarding a safety plan and establishing care with a therapist. At the end of the visit, you ask the student to reflect on the visit. They recall the specific eating disorder behaviors you asked the patient about, and you discuss the meaning of "body checking," a term with which they were unfamiliar. You also ask the student to reflect on the language and communication strategies they observed you utilizing. You have a longer discussion about higher levels of care for mental health and disordered eating and discuss criteria for hospital admission for medical stabilization. The student expresses appreciation for having had the benefit of discretely listening in on and learning from the visit without feeling intrusive.

Key Takeaway Points

Actively engaging learners in telehealth encounters even when they are non-participatory observers can be a highly valuable educational tool. If acceptable to the patient, sensitive telehealth visits can be silently observed by learners in a way that may be less obtrusive than shadowing an in-person visit.

Strengths and Limitations of Telehealth in Medical Training

Clinical teaching through telehealth has its advantages and disadvantages both to the learner and to the preceptor. Throughout the COVID-19 pandemic, while students and trainees were initially sent home and excluded from clinical care to prevent the spread of infection often in the setting of inadequate supply of personal protective equipment, telehealth served as a means to rapidly reincorporate learners of all levels in a safe way [4]. Trainees have reported a benefit of convenience and flexibility, with no need to commute to work if able to access telehealth platforms from home [21]. Telehealth also allows learners to see adolescents in their home environments where they may be more at ease, often open to incorporating their pets or hobbies into the visit; this may serve as a unique means to better understand adolescent development for the learner. Without the ability to perform a physical exam, remote clinical encounters have shifted clinicians and learners to focus more on the "lost art" of collecting a detailed history, a crucial skill for medical learners [25]. Trainees also benefit from direct observation by their attendings, as well as the ability to actively observe others in a virtual setting. Receiving subsequent real-time feedback on their performance in the clinical encounter is an advantage perceived as highly valuable by most learners [17, 21]. Benefits of efficiency have also been reported, including ability for trainees to complete timely documentation and ability for attending physician to complete notes from a prior visit while listening in on trainee's interview, when appropriate.

One of the challenges of telehealth specific to clinical education includes difficulty for preceptors to model rapport-building with adolescents via a virtual platform. Similarly, trainees may have concerns about or struggle with developing a connection with teens virtually. The inability to ensure complete confidentiality in their homes may also be a barrier for some youth in feeling at ease in sharing questions or concerns with the learner. While there are also challenges with an in-person visit that entails wearing a mask that conceals facial expressions, some youth may be less receptive to engaging with new providers including trainees in a virtual setting. Additionally, the inability to obtain measurements and vital signs and the lack of physical exam are major disadvantages of telehealth-based learning [26]. Teaching trainees to identify vital sign instability or clinical signs of malnutrition (e.g., lanugo, acrocyanosis) in a patient with anorexia nervosa (see Chap. 8 on eating disorder care) is an important skill in adolescent medicine. These strengths and limitations are summarized in Table 5.2.

Table 5.2 Advantages and disadvantages of telehealth in adolescent medicine clinical education [21]

Advantages	Disadvantages
Infection prevention	Connectivity/technology failures
Convenience, flexibility	Challenging to develop rapport-building
No commute	skills virtually with youth
Allows learners to see adolescents in their home environments	Learner discomfort regarding threats to adolescent confidentiality
Ability for learners to observe patients' facial expression, without a mask	Lack of physical exam skill teaching
Ability to receive direct observation from preceptor	
Efficiency with trainee and preceptor documentation	

Impact of Telehealth on Clinical Training

With the COVID-19 pandemic affecting most aspects of graduate medical education (GME), it is critical to understand the immediate and longer-term impacts this had had on medical trainees throughout the nation. One study conducted by the Accreditation Council for Graduate Medical Education (ACGME) looked at program directors' responses to a COVID-19 supplement as part of their 2021 annual program updates. This study reported on data from 11,250 GME programs of all disciplines and specialties. More than half of specialty programs that included ambulatory continuity clinics reported a decline in overall training opportunities during the pandemic, and 42.1% of programs reported significant disruption due to COVID-19 for 1–6 months of training. Forty percent of programs used telehealth for up to 25% of patient encounters, 14.1% of programs used it 25–49% of the time, 9% used it 50–74% of the time, and 9.5% used it 75% or more of patient encounters [27]. Given this rapidly expanding area of clinical care, the Association of American Medical Colleges (AAMC) has subsequently announced that telemedicine will become one of the "entrustable professional activities" (EPA) that medical students must learn moving forward [27].

Another study sought to assess the prevalence of telemedicine experiences in internal medicine (IM) core clerkships for medical students before and after the start of the pandemic. This national survey of IM clerkship directors found that, despite the ability to return to in-person clinical care once the acute phase of the pandemic had subsided, the use of telehealth continued intentionally, suggesting the perceived value of telehealth as an effective educational tool during the clerkship. This study also found that clerkship directors within programs having a significant ambulatory component reported perceiving telehealth as an important competency, whereas clerkship directors from programs with predominant focus on inpatient care regarded it as less valuable, possibly due to telehealth being more challenging to replicate in the inpatient setting [28].

To date, there are very few studies exploring perspectives of the learners themselves regarding use of telemedicine and its impact on their medical education. One small study surveyed trainees rotating through an adolescent medicine specialty clinic and found that the majority of trainees (83.3%) rated their educational experience with telehealth as either effective or very effective, and among trainees who had exposure to a greater number of telehealth sessions during their rotation, all reported telehealth as effective or very effective mode of clinical teaching. All trainees in the study reported interest in incorporating telehealth into their future practice [23]. Another recent study describes a needs assessment of a family medicine residency program in the U.S. comparing perceived self-confidence in faculty assessment and resident performance of select telehealth clinical skills. Both trainees and faculty reported comfort with telehealth clinical skills but identified a need for better teaching of virtual communication and physical exam skills during video visits [29]. Further research in this field will be needed to better understand the long-term impact of trainee experiences in remote clinical learning and to identify unmet educational gaps.

Telehealth Curricula in Medical Education

An emerging body of literature reports on the presence of and attempts at implementation of telehealth curricula across undergraduate and graduate medical education in the U.S. since the pandemic began. In one study, leaders in undergraduate medical education from eight different disciplines were surveyed to determine changes in telehealth curriculum for medical students, finding that the majority of programs (81%) had no formal training in telehealth prior to the pandemic, but only 3% reported no training after the pandemic onset. Faculty identified competing curricular demands (29%) and lack of faculty training (22%) as the greatest barriers to teaching telehealth at their medical schools [30].

Another study looked at the administration of an asynchronous five-module telemedicine curriculum at Harvard Medical School focusing on knowledge and skills required to conduct live video encounters. Comparison of pre- and post-course surveys revealed an increase in students' self-rated knowledge of telemedicine from 15.1% being fairly or very knowledgeable over four domains prior to the course to 84.3% after conclusion of the course. The majority of students (85.9%) reported that the course met their learning needs and most (81.5%) found the delivery methods to be effective [31].

Telehealth curricula have also been integrated into residency training at some institutions. One such example is a pilot study conducted at Cohen Children's Medical Center/Zucker School of Medicine at Hofstra-Northwell in New York with pediatric interns during their orientation week. Interns first participated and were observed in a mock ambulatory video encounter on Zoom to "practice" telemedicine skills. The intervention group was then asked to review materials of a telemedicine curriculum, while the control group was not. Both groups were again observed in a mock Zoom patient encounter the following week. Results demonstrated a statistically significant improvement in total communication scores of interns who completed the telehealth curriculum, particularly in categories of privacy assurance, rapport establishment, demonstration of empathy, and partnership building [7].

While many medical training programs have begun to incorporate telehealth curricula, they are often not mandatory for students and trainees, and even for those who do offer this, there are no formal guidelines regarding content. Leaders in medical education have called for a change in future curricula, including instruction on the legal, ethical, and regulatory components of telehealth [32]. There is also a need for more formalized studies to evaluate best practices for teaching telehealth to the next generation of physicians.

Summary

The ever-changing field of medicine is reliant upon the education of students and trainees to ensure continued advancement and innovation in clinical practice. The COVID-19 pandemic has threatened traditional models for clinical education yet has presented opportunities for novel and engaging teaching methodologies. Telehealth has not only permitted medical trainees to observe and play an active role in caring for patients remotely during the COVID-19 pandemic but may also afford unique educational benefits not available through traditional in-person clinical teaching [6, 21, 33]. Telemedicine is now considered a vital component of clinical care, and while learners have contributed valuable suggestions from their perspectives as digital natives [5], leaders in medical education have a duty to continue to evaluate and refine our teaching skills through this modality to improve the quality of training moving forward. A positive, supportive telehealth experience during medical school and residency may increase trainees' willingness to provide this care in the future, thus investing in training infrastructure and reimagining the role of virtual care may be of value. Medical educators have argued for a shift from use of telehealth as a direct replacement for in-person instruction to instead taking advantage of unique aspects to reinvent and enhance education [34]. The pandemic has provided us new opportunities to reimagine and transform medical training, yet there is need for further studies to investigate best practices and establish clear guidelines for tele-precepting. There is no question that telehealth will continue to be a significant part of trainees' careers moving forward; our actions and innovations today in implementing curricula can support a positive legacy of the COVID-19 pandemic on medical education of the future.

References

1. Evans YN, et al. Using telemedicine to reach adolescents during the COVID-19 pandemic. J Adolesc Health. 2020;67(4):469–71.
2. Emans SJ, et al. Early COVID-19 impact on adolescent health and medicine programs in the United States: LEAH program leadership reflections. J Adolesc Health. 2020;67(1):11–5.
3. Muntz MD, et al. Telehealth and medical student education in the time of COVID-19-and beyond. Acad Med. 2021;96(12):1655–9.
4. Gallagher TH, Schleyer AM. "We signed up for this!"—student and trainee responses to the Covid-19 pandemic. N Engl J Med. 2020;382(25):e96.
5. Pathipati AS, Azad TD, Jethwani K. Telemedical education: training digital natives in telemedicine. J Med Internet Res. 2016;18(7):e193.
6. Klasen JM, et al. "The storm has arrived": the impact of SARS-CoV-2 on medical students. Perspect Med Educ. 2020;9(3):181–5.

7. Samuels R, et al. Cultivating "webside manner" at the UME-GME transition point during the COVID-19 pandemic: a novel virtual telemedicine curriculum. J Med Educat Curri Develop. 2022;9:23821205221096361.
8. Pourmand A, et al. Lack of telemedicine training in academic medicine: are we preparing the next generation? Telemed J E Health. 2020;27:62.
9. Ho PA, et al. Advancing medical education through innovations in teaching during the COVID-19 pandemic. Prim Care Companion CNS Disord. 2021;23(1)
10. Said JT, Schwartz AW. Remote medical education: adapting Kern's curriculum design to tele-teaching. Med Sci Educ. 2021;31(2):805–12.
11. Erlich D, Armstrong E, Gooding H. Silver linings: a thematic analysis of case studies describing advances in health professions education during the COVID-19 pandemic. Med Teach. 2021;43(12):1444–9.
12. Shaterjalali M, Changiz T, Yamani N. Optimal clinical setting, tutors, and learning opportunities in medical education: a content analysis. (2277-9531 (Print)).
13. Dedeilia A, et al. Medical and surgical education challenges and innovations in the COVID-19 era: a systematic review. In Vivo. 2020;34(3 Suppl):1603–11.
14. Chick RC, et al. Using technology to maintain the education of residents during the COVID-19 pandemic. J Surg Educ. 2020;77(4):729–32.
15. Oldenburg R, Marsch A. Optimizing teledermatology visits for dermatology resident education during the COVID-19 pandemic. J Am Acad Dermatol. 2020;82(6):e229.
16. Koumpouras F, Helfgott S. Stand together and deliver: challenges and opportunities for rheumatology education during the COVID-19 pandemic. Arthritis Rheumatol. 2020;72(7):1064–6.
17. Pellegrini WR, Danis DO 3rd, Levi JR. Medical student participation in otolaryngology telemedicine clinic during COVID-19: a hidden opportunity. Otolaryngol Head Neck Surg. 2021;164(6):1131–3.
18. Erlich D. The triumph of teleteaching: tips for incorporating students into outpatient tele-medicine. Webinar. Tufts University School of Medicine, Office of Continuing Medical Education; 2020.
19. Erlich D. Triangle method: teaching the student in front of the patient. Acad Med. 2019;94(4):605.
20. Mittal V. Family-centered rounds. Pediatr Clin N Am. 2014;61(4):663–70.
21. Golub SA, et al. Evaluating the educational impact of telehealth on adolescent medicine trainees: a qualitative approach. Curr Pediatr Rep. 2021;9:72–6.
22. Hovaguimian A, et al. Twelve tips for clinical teaching with telemedicine visits. Med Teach. 2022;44(1):19–25.
23. Pham DQ, et al. The impact of telehealth on clinical education in adolescent medicine during the COVID-19 pandemic: positive preliminary findings. Front Pediatr. 2021;9:642279.
24. Gardner AL, et al. Huddling for high-performing teams. Fed Pract. 2018;35(9):16–22.
25. Wijesooriya NR, et al. COVID-19 and telehealth, education, and research adaptations. Paediatr Respir Rev. 2020;35:38–42.
26. Woolliscroft JO. Innovation in response to the COVID-19 pandemic crisis. Acad Med. 2020;95(8):1140–2.
27. Hogan SO, Holmboe ES. Effects of COVID-19 on residency and fellowship training: results of a national survey. J Grad Med Educ. 2022;14(3):359–64.
28. Henschen BL, et al. Teaching telemedicine in the COVID-19 era: a National Survey of Internal Medicine Clerkship Directors. J Gen Intern Med. 2021;36(11):3497–502.
29. Venditti SA, et al. Family medicine resident and faculty perceptions about the strengths and limitations of telemedicine training. PRiMER. 2022;6:9.
30. Jortberg BT, et al. Expansion of telehealth curriculum: national survey of clinical education leaders. J Telemed Telecare. 2022;28(6):464–8.

31. Frankl SE, et al. Preparing future doctors for telemedicine: an asynchronous curriculum for medical students implemented during the COVID-19 pandemic. Acad Med. 2021;96(12):1696–701.
32. Jumreornvong O, et al. Telemedicine and medical education in the age of COVID-19. Acad Med. 2020;95(12):1838–43.
33. Rasmussen S, et al. Medical students for health-care staff shortages during the COVID-19 pandemic. Lancet. 2020;395(10234):e79–80.
34. Anderson HL, et al. Replace, amplify, transform: a qualitative study of how postgraduate trainees and supervisors experience and use telehealth for instruction in ambulatory patient care. BMC Med Educ. 2022;22(1):118.

Chapter 6
Telemedicine Use in Adolescent Primary Care

Ellen Bryant, Laura Dos Reis, and Emily Ruedinger

Introduction

Telemedicine has become an important tool in the medical care of adolescents, especially as virtual interactions became ubiquitous during the COVID-19 pandemic. Telemedicine encourages social distancing and decreases patient exposure to medical facilities, which are important benefits during a pandemic. There are other benefits as well related to convenience and efficiency [1]. Telemedicine eliminates the need for travel to appointments, which leads to increased access to healthcare, especially in rural or underserved populations (see equity (Chap. 3), rural health (Chap. 4), gender care (Chap. 11), and justice involved youth (Chap. 12) as examples). The time saved traveling to appointments equates to fewer missed work hours for parents or caregivers. In fact, a study by McConnochie found that children had an average of over 4 fewer absences per 100 school days with telehealth appointments [2]. Telemedicine may also improve monitoring of medical issues, as well as reduce unnecessary emergency room visits [3].

Telemedicine has been well received by patients and families and may actually be preferred by adolescents who generally are comfortable using electronic devices. A study by Fleischman et al. compared in-person physician visits to a combination of in-person and telemedicine visits in the treatment of children with obesity. They found that the majority of patients included in the study, as well as their parents, would choose telemedicine visits over in-person visits moving forward [4].

E. Bryant (✉)
Children's Mercy Hospital, Kansas City, MO, USA

L. D. Reis · E. Ruedinger
University of Wisconsin, Madison, WI, USA
e-mail: ldosreis@uwhealth.org; eruedinger@wisc.edu

© The Author(s), under exclusive license to Springer Nature
Switzerland AG 2024
Y. N. Evans et al. (eds.), *Telemedicine for Adolescent and Young Adult Health Care*, https://doi.org/10.1007/978-3-031-55760-6_6

Ramaswamy et al. noted a slight, but statistically significant, increase in satisfaction scores from patients in regard to telemedicine over traditional, in-person visits [5].

Most importantly, telemedicine has been shown to deliver equal or even superior care as compared to in-person visits in certain situations. There have been a variety of studies comparing telemedicine to in-person visits which suggest that telemedicine visits are especially helpful for medical issues which require longitudinal care over multiple follow-up visits, such as in asthma and type I diabetes [6–8].

It is important to acknowledge the limitations of telemedicine, including inability to perform a full physical exam, obtain labs or other testing, or provide immediate treatments or vaccines. The limitations of telemedicine will be explored later in this chapter (see section "Limitations"). Reassuringly, telemedicine can be used to effectively triage patients with an acute concern. A study by Siew et al. found that telemedicine visits could reliably recognize patients that were seriously ill [9]. Ideally, a provider would be able to recognize an ill patient and refer them to be seen in person. On the other hand, for patients who are less ill and may require only further monitoring or supportive care at home, a provider may be able to save a patient a potentially costly and time-consuming emergency department visit with the use of telemedicine.

Prior to the Telemedicine Visit

Develop a Workflow

Your clinic should first establish a workflow surrounding telemedicine visits. There is no one perfect workflow, as each community, clinic, and health record may vary. In general, it is ideal for patients to receive the information on how to log on to the telemedicine visit a few days prior. This may be done electronically with contact information for troubleshooting, or via telephone for patients who may need assistance setting up their technology. There should be some means of confirming the visit and that the patient has appropriate technology, whether electronic, automated, direct call from office staff, or otherwise. At the time of the visit, the medical assistant may be the first to join the virtual space to confirm patient information, ask routine screening questions, and collect vitals (see section "Vital Signs") [10]. Gusdorf et al. noted that structured pre-visit phone calls are also associated with a higher likelihood of a successful virtual visit [11].

When the medical assistant is done, they should be able to communicate through a flag, color-coded symbol, or secure message that the patient is ready to be seen by a provider. Your patient may also need to be seen by another staff member to receive additional teaching or resources (such as nursing staff providing asthma teaching or social workers providing resources). This may also be the case for multidisciplinary clinics. If so, the staff member should be able to join the virtual space after you complete your visit to proceed with their part. Eliminating or minimizing the need for the patient to log in/log out, or switch virtual rooms, is ideal. It is important to consider how staff members participating in the visit will communicate with each other. Some electronic health records may have a "secure chat" feature, which may be an ideal way to communicate. There should also be a clear process by which follow-up visits are arranged.

Set the Stage

Choose a location for your workstation that is private and quiet. The location should be well lit, and your background should be simple. If feasible, set up your video monitor so that anyone interrupting the encounter cannot view the patient.

Ensure that your camera, speakers, and microphone are all working. Consider using headphones to improve privacy if conversations are easily overhead at your workstation. Take a look at how you will appear to your patient beforehand. Ideally, you should sit close enough to the camera so that your face and about half your torso is visible. Choose professional attire and wear your medical badge so that it is visible to the camera [12, 13].

Just prior to beginning the visit, secure the room by closing the door. You may also want to put up a sign that says "Virtual visit in progress" to discourage accidental interruptions.

Starting the Visit

First, ensure that the patient is not experiencing any technical difficulties. Confirm that they can see and hear you [1]. Introduce yourself and confirm the identity of the patient and anyone else present in the visit. Be sure to look directly at your camera to simulate eye contact and not down at the image of the patient [1]. We suggest confirming the patient's phone number and current location at the start of the visit, in case of technical issues or emergencies. This may also be pertinent to ensure you are appropriately licensed to provide care for the patient in their current location based on state laws. It is also important to confirm that your patient is joining the call from a safe location. If your patient is joining the call from an unsafe location, such as while driving, ask if they can pull over. If they are unable to, end the visit and have a scheduler or other support staff call back at a later time to reschedule the visit. Similarly, if the patient is not in a private location, assess for their willingness to continue versus reschedule. You may suggest they use headphones for added privacy if they are available to the patient.

We have found that adolescents may often present to telemedicine visits on their own, whether at school, work, or home alone. It is important to confirm whether a parent is available to consent to any medical treatment and, if not, how to get in contact with a parent. Adolescents are able to consent to some medical care themselves. Guidelines vary by state, with youth often being able to consent to some or all of the following medical care: mental healthcare, substance use, treatment of sexually transmitted infections, and reproductive healthcare [14]. Consent can be presumed for emergency medical treatment for which delay may cause the patient serious harm, such as calling an ambulance for a patient with severe respiratory distress [15].

Vital Signs

You are likely accustomed to reviewing a set of vitals prior to beginning an in-person clinic visit. Although vital signs are more difficult to obtain in a virtual visit, it is possible to have your patient report their own vital signs with the use of digital devices [16]. Your patient may own a smartwatch which can measure pulse (and it may even be able to obtain a limited EKG). Some patients may also own a blood pressure cuff, thermometer, and a scale. It may be helpful to include a reminder for the patient to have digital devices on hand at their telemedicine visit and to incorporate vital sign collection into the workflow of the medical assistant who is first to meet with the patient in the virtual space.

Technological advances may further enhance the virtual physical exam. For instance, there are otoscopes that can be connected to a smartphone for parents to photograph their child's tympanic membrane. However, more studies are needed to determine the reliability and usefulness of the smartphone otoscope in practice, and access is currently limited [17].

Well Visit

Per AAP guidance, it remains strongly recommended that well-child care occurs in person when feasible. When this is not possible, they recommend telemedicine be followed by a timely in-person visit and examination [18]. Several studies have shown that, when necessary, many annual well visits in adolescents, including those for chronic disease management, can be completed over telemedicine [19–21]. When surveying physicians providing telemedicine in the early months of the COVID-19 pandemic, Gilkey et al. found that the majority of providers seeing adolescents virtually were doing so for chronic disease management, acute care, behavioral and mental health concerns, and vaccine consultations, with fewer providing other forms of well care [22]. Similarly, Barney et al. also initially did not offer virtual well visits [19]. As the COVID-19 pandemic went on, they and many other institutions have been able to incorporate many of the valuable elements of well care into the practice of telemedicine [19, 22].

In order to facilitate a more complete and efficient visit, it is recommended you use questionnaires in the same way you would with an in-person visit. This would include standardized screens, such as the Patient Health Questionnaire-9 (PHQ-9) and Generalized Anxiety Disorder-7 (GAD-7), as well as your institution's typical before-visit paperwork [23, 24]. As we will discuss further below, patient surveys not only streamline the visit, but they have also been associated with improved patient recall of anticipatory guidance and with improved clinician counseling [25, 26]. It is also a benefit of telemedicine that patients can review their medication list with the pill bottles, which can be helpful to assess what is truly being taken, what dosages they have, and what supplements they are taking without relying on their memory [27].

Your clinic may accomplish this in several ways. Some clinics do so by utilizing medical assistants to work through questionnaires during the patient check-in process. It is also possible to send them in advance, through a patient portal, mail, or other means. Ideally, completion of forms in a patient portal that directly links to the patient electronic medical record (EMR) is most efficient. As more clinics and institutions migrate to technology-assisted appointment check-in, this process becomes easier to translate to telemedicine. Patients may upload forms via email, though this is an insecure form of information sharing for patient data and is generally not recommended. Patients could be asked to submit a picture of the paperwork to the chart, similar to a picture of a concern, if no other means for uploading questionnaires are available within your institution. Special considerations around confidentiality and timing of mental health screening, such as provision of questions containing time-sensitive information like suicide screening, are covered in the chapter on mental health.

All well visits should continue to include age-appropriate screening regarding topics such as food insecurity, dental care, vision, school performance, safety, depression, substance use, abuse, trafficking risk, and others. Providers remain mandated reporters, regardless of visit type [28]. This may be accomplished via a thorough HEADSSS exam. When indicated, appropriate screening laboratory work should be ordered. Many clinics provide free barrier protection along with safe sex counseling. If this service will not be provided to patients via alternative means (i.e., mailing all patients condoms), it would be useful to provide patients with a list of community sites with free or low-cost barrier protection, if available in your area.

H Home: caregivers, other persons in the home, time spent with each caregiver (if multiple homes), support, conflicts

E Education: grade level, performance, difficult subjects, difficulty seeing or hearing, bullying, concentration, attendance, future plans

A Activities: sports, club participation, hobbies, friends/peer support, screen time, physical activity, employment

D Drugs: substance use (type, quantity, frequency), secondhand exposure, desire to quit/cut down use, use with driving or other high-risk situations

D Diet: typical foods/meals, special diet (i.e. vegan), difficulties with eating, food availability, body image and any steps taken to change appearance

S Sexuality: gender identity, partner gender preferences, history/types of sexual activity, plans to become sexually active, number/gender of current/former partners, use of barriers and other contraceptives, pregnancy, STIs

S Suicidality: prior or current suicidal ideation (including passive thoughts), self-harm history, mood, anxiety/worry, sadness/depression

S Safety: safety in home/school/relationship/neighborhood, history of physical/emotional/sexual abuse, storage of potentially harmful objects at home

While it is not feasible to complete several important examination requirements of a sports physical virtually (cardiac, pulmonary, lymph nodes, and others requiring palpation or auscultation), one may utilize telemedicine to limit the length of in-person visit required, to avoid delays in well care, and to increase overall access to care. Additionally, several aspects of the physical exam can and should be incorporated over telemedicine if the patient will not be able to schedule a timely in-person physical evaluation. These will likely be performed in only a limited capacity: mobility/functional testing through double-leg squat testing, abdominal exam, musculoskeletal exam, scoliosis screening, skin examination, and other exams as feasible. Screening blood pressures yearly for adolescents is recommended by the American Academy of Pediatrics and especially important for patients on stimulants, steroids, tricyclic antidepressants, or hormonal contraceptives [29]. If patients have access to a home blood pressure cuff of appropriate size, it is recommended that you ask them to utilize it, in addition to checking blood pressure at their next in-person appointment. Routine screening of sensitive exam areas for sexual maturity rating may be uncomfortable for some patients or providers to perform in the virtual environment. Sensitive exams are suggested to be performed only if the patient and provider are comfortable. Several studies have shown fair ability of children and adolescents to self-report current sexual maturity rating [30, 31]. You may choose to show pictures and descriptions and ask patients to self-categorize their current breast and genital development. Of note, accuracy is improved when patients are provided with both pictures and descriptions, as well as for those who are at either end of the development spectrum (either early/pre-puberty or late/post-puberty) [30]. Please see the section "Virtual Physical Exam" later in this chapter for more detailed guidance.

Transition of care to adult medical providers should continue to be performed regardless of visit type. Virtual visits may even offer advantages over traditional in-person transfers of care, as it may be possible for both the pediatric and adult provider to be present for the visit. You should continue to use a formal transition policy, discuss transition early and often, plan transitions, and follow-up afterward [32, 33].

Case: Well Visit

Jess, a 17-year-old, non-binary (assigned female at birth) teen who uses they/them/ theirs pronouns is seen for their annual well visit. They are seen over telemedicine after school and live about 15 min from the clinic. Due to their school schedule early in the year, they did not want to miss school for their appointment, so requested to have it over telemedicine. They have a history of exercise-induced asthma but have needed their albuterol very rarely over the past year. They are seen initially with their father, who logs in separately from work and reports no concerns. After a brief discussion, he logs off to allow Jess privacy. They have been doing well since their last visit and have no specific concerns today. They have no significant health history and take no regular medications.

They have been growing and developing well previously, now with stable self-reported height. When you plot the weight they reported to the medical assistant prior to joining the visit, you note they are gaining weight along their prior percentile. The heart rate and respiratory rate that Jess reports are within normal limits for age. They do not have a home blood pressure cuff, so no further vital signs are available.

They play basketball and are interested in having their annual sports physical form signed, though the season will not start for 2 months. You discuss options for this, noting that you can perform the majority of the visit virtually, but will need to see them in person for a physical exam prior to signing their physical form.

They do note that they are bothered by having their period. They are currently sexually active with their boyfriend. Menses started 4 years ago. Periods are regular with light to moderate bleeding and mild cramps at the start of each period. They have not noticed issues with mood or other symptoms around periods. They have not had previous partners and report no concerns for symptoms of a sexually transmitted infection. They have exclusively penile-vaginal sex and use an external condom with every sexual encounter. You discuss the gamut of contraception. Jess would like to start the depot medroxyprogesterone acetate injection. You also provide them with trustworthy resources for additional research on methods.

They filled out the PHQ-9 and GAD-7 through the patient portal prior to starting the visit. They report no concerns with their mood and deny feelings of sadness or worry. Their affect appears consistent with this. They report no history of self-harm, suicidal ideation, or suicide attempts. Their screenings show low concern for both anxiety and depression, similar to their prior screen results. They are doing well in school and there are no concerns about body image or substance use when discussing this further. You provide general anticipatory guidance to Jess, including substance use, relationships, reproductive health, and safety. They do report recreational screen time of 4 h daily, up from 1 h daily at their last visit.

Acknowledging the irony of discussing increased screen time with them through a screen, you use motivational interviewing techniques to discuss the reasons behind their increased screen time, as well as potential options to decrease this. They volunteer that they used to enjoy biking with friends and playing Dungeons and Dragons, but that this stopped at the start of the COVID-19 pandemic. After discussing further, they decide to try to do both with friends each week.

A virtual physical exam is performed, using methods discussed later in this chapter. Jess's father rejoins the visit to discuss the plan for their next visit and topics discussed today. They plan to set up a brief appointment in the coming month, to include blood pressure measurement, the remainder of the physical exam, a depot medroxyprogesterone acetate shot, their annual influenza vaccination, and to have their sports physical form signed. They also plan to visit the laboratory to obtain screening non-fasting lipids, as well as routine gonorrhea and chlamydia screening. You refill their albuterol prescription and go over an updated asthma action plan with them. You provide an after-visit summary that discusses your anticipatory guidance, screening recommendations, asthma action plan, and anticipated well-care needs. You walk Jess and their father through how to obtain it from the patient portal.

The appointment allowed Jess to discuss their mental and physical well-being and afforded them the opportunity to begin lifestyle changes. Overall, things were going very well for this patient, though certainly this visit could have allowed you to pick up on concerning new physical or mental concerns to prompt an even sooner in-person visit.

They were able to discuss their chronic disease management and have their prescription refilled. Even though they were not able to accomplish their main goals for the visit today (have their sports physical signed and improve periods), they did have the opportunity to make a plan for both of these, as well as limit the amount of in-office time that will be required at their next appointment. They are afforded time to research and consider their contraceptive choice without the burden of two in-person appointments. They did not have to drive straight to the office from school or miss school for their appointment today. Their father was able to join, even though he was still at work. Their upcoming visit for their exam, vitals, vaccine, injection, and lab work can be far shorter than a typical well visit and may have them miss less school overall [34].

Not all patients will have a home scale and be able to report a current weight nor does that assure it is accurate. Trending weight can be a helpful guide, but we recommend you discuss healthy lifestyle goals and changes with all patients, regardless of their weight or body mass index (BMI). Not only does this reduce bias and feelings of shame for patients, but it also allows you to focus on potential changes identified by patients. Using motivational interviewing to explore health habits increases the likelihood that goals are helpful and sustainable [35]. A study by Matheson et al. showed significant improvements in mortality with lifestyle habit changes, regardless of changes in patient weight or BMI [36].

Anticipatory Guidance

It is recommended you give anticipatory guidance much in the same way as an in-person visit. There is the potential added benefit that there may be ways to tailor this guidance based on findings noted in the patient home when video visits are attended from the home. Shenkman et al. found that one quarter of providers appreciate the telehealth benefit of anticipatory guidance tailored to the visualized home environment. As with all teenage visits, it is important to provide teens with privacy and time to discuss questions and concerns alone with their provider. While evidence is limited, Shenkman et al. suggest anticipatory guidance may be more impactful when providers have one-on-one time in teen visits. Though current telemedicine research is even more sparse, it stands to reason those similar principles apply, and it may be more impactful to provide anticipatory guidance at times in the visit when the teen has privacy. This also ensures that provided guidance can be pertinent after questionnaire completion and/or a discussion of risk behaviors regarding health maintenance (screen time, diet, activity), social-emotional health, substance use, personal safety, and sexual health.

Additional considerations may be needed when providing anticipatory guidance to teens with various disabilities and chronic illnesses [37]. Please ensure that you take additional time to explore these concerns as needed, noting that to do so may require screening separate from typical questionnaires and screeners, as well as more targeted recommendations. It is important to provide typical adolescent risk-behavior counseling and screening regarding health behaviors in a way that is developmentally appropriate [37]. All adolescent patients deserve an opportunity for privacy with their providers, and every effort to provide this should be made. Additionally, it is recommended that you take extra care to discuss several topics. Maintaining an active lifestyle can look differently for teens with disabilities. It may be overlooked in typical screening or not assessed due to an assumption of a sedentary lifestyle for such individuals. For counseling regarding activity level, discuss barriers, include modifications as necessary, and include specific advice and guidance to help all teens stay or become appropriately active [37].

Children with disabilities may also be at higher risk of social isolation, concomitant mental health challenges, and stress [37]. Adequately addressing this may require more specialized referrals and knowledge of social groups and local resources, which can be very beneficial for patients. Additional attention should also be provided regarding dental care, which can also be more challenging; home oral care, preventative care, and treatment should be discussed or provided by practitioners with experience working with teens with disabilities [37]. In addition, teens with disabilities are at higher risk for abuse and violence; remain vigilant for signs of abuse in all teens, recognizing that concerns may manifest differently over telemedicine [28, 38].

Motivational interviewing is one of the briefest techniques to employ an evidence-based behavioral intervention, as compared to other psychosocial approaches [39]. Therefore, it is often the method of choice utilized by providers when discussing changing health behaviors during well and problem visits. Motivational interviewing has shown improvements in substance use reduction, medication adherence, dietary and activity changes, as well as many other lifestyle changes [39–41]. Several studies have shown that using motivational interviewing techniques over telemedicine remains efficacious [35, 40–43].

Concern Visits

There are several primary concerns that lend themselves well to telemedicine due to their limited need for significant physical examination. However, many of these concerns are also more emotional topics to broach with teens. While some adolescents may appreciate the convenience and other benefits of telehealth, and perhaps even welcome the physical separation from providers when discussing emotional topics, others may express a preference to discuss these topics in person, either initially or indefinitely [44, 45]. Allowing patients and their families to choose their preferred visit type, within reason, is the best way to maximize patients' sense of ownership over their health and overall patient-centered care [46, 47]. Overall, video visits have been shown to be preferable to voice-only visits [47].

As with an in-person visit, it is important to be transparent regarding any learners involved in the appointment, as well as if any portion of the visit will be recorded for research or other purposes [48, 49].

One study found that despite 98% of teens identifying that they utilized a private space to conduct visits from home, only 78% of that group was comfortable with the level of visit privacy [50]. In order to facilitate feelings of security and privacy, you should utilize HIPAA-compliant telemedicine platforms and a secure Internet connection for increased web security. All participants in the call, including those in the same room as the provider, should be introduced [49]. Some teens may be more comfortable if they are able to see the entire room or office from which the provider is conducting the visit. Concern for not knowing who is in the room was cited as another privacy concern [50]. When you or the teen are unable to ensure visit privacy, you can promote privacy by encouraging headphone usage, using yes/no questions, or utilizing the chat function [51]. Open-ended discussions regarding teen preference for visit type when feasible may help to ensure visits are comfortable and productive.

Presuming patients are comfortable being seen over telemedicine, concerns that are most conducive to a virtual visit include mental health complaints, sleep issues, acne, contraception counseling, and menstrual issues [19, 51]. Please see the respective chapters elsewhere in this book for more detailed information regarding reproductive health and mental health. Of note, the Ryan Haight Online Pharmacy Consumer Protection Act of 2008 does allow for prescribing of controlled substances over telemedicine, but patients must have been evaluated at least once in person previously [49]. This is important to keep in mind for attention deficit disorder and attention deficit hyperactivity disorder visits. Other visit concerns are much more difficult, if not impossible to do over telemedicine. Others still are accomplished only when able to recommend adjunct laboratory or imaging studies to be performed.

Some teens with medical complexity or other concerns may have home support devices. These same patients may also be at highest risk for exposure to illness at an in-person clinic visit. It may be more difficult to come into the office due to physical distance from the clinic or transportation issues, like any patient, but this can be especially complicated when adaptive transportation is required. For these reasons and simply family preference, virtual visits may be ideal for home medical equipment malfunction (such as nasogastric tubes, central lines, or other devices), as you can go through home troubleshooting, as well as have them demonstrate the typical home care provided [27].

Visits for headaches, asthma, or constipation can all be reasonably performed, though would be more complete with an in-person examination in the clinic [19]. Follow-up visits for these concerns would be better suited to virtual visits than initial presentations.

Acute orthopedic complaints, need for STI screening, and concern for a urinary tract infection are all visits that can be performed over telemedicine while instructing the patient and potentially a caregiver in key physical exam maneuvers. However, these visits require that the patient be able to access laboratory screening or imaging if necessary to form a more complete diagnosis and treatment plan. A study by Wilson et al. suggests virtual referral for STI screening, even in an automated fashion, may increase the percentage of teens who perform STI screening [52]. Some concerns may be possible to address only if labs provide testing more commonly performed by providers, such as throat streptococcal or STI screening. Vaginal discharge complaints are unlikely to be fully evaluated virtually unless self-swabs (including wet mount preparation and KOH testing) are available.

Virtual Physical Exam

Your goal should be to deliver the same quality of care virtually as compared to in-person. It is therefore important to practice techniques to optimize the virtual physical exam. Here, you will find an approach to the virtual physical exam.

Beginning the Physical Exam

You may remember receiving the advice during your medical training, "your physical exam begins the moment you walk into the patient's room." Similarly, the physical exam of a virtual visit begins when your patient first appears on screen. In the first few moments of the virtual visit, you will be able to observe the patient's general appearance, work of breathing, body language, mood/affect, and any visible skin findings. Depending on where your patient is joining the telemedicine visit, you may also be able to observe your patient's living situation or work/school environment. You may also be able to observe interactions between your patient and their family members or significant others if they are also present at the visit or in the background. Providers have even observed intimate partner violence during telemedicine visits [53]. For mental health visits, the state of your patient's living space may give you insight into how they are doing. In this way, telemedicine can give you unique insight into a patient's behaviors, environment, and social circumstances which would not be possible in traditional in-person clinic visits.

Before you begin your physical exam, explain to the patient that because you are meeting virtually, you will need their help in performing the physical exam. Throughout the exam, explain to the patient what you are doing and give them clear instructions of what you would like them to do.

Guide for Performing a Telemedicine Physical Exam [16]

Skin

Have the patient take a picture of their skin and upload it to the patient portal prior to the appointment. You can have your patient perform a skin "self-assessment" and show you any new rashes or moles.

HEENT

Has your patient noticed any changes to vision or hearing? You can observe pupil symmetry, scleral icterus, or conjunctival injection. You may also be able to observe other findings, such as ptosis. Ask your patient to swallow. Did they experience any pain with swallowing? Ask your patient to turn their head and look over their right shoulder and then their left shoulder. Did they experience any pain or stiffness? While they are moving their neck, observe their range of motion.

Lung

Have your patient take a deep breath. Did you hear any coughing, stridor, or wheezing? You can observe their respiratory rate and whether they are experiencing any increased work of breathing.

Cardiac

The cardiac exam is understandably limited in the virtual setting. Digital devices, such as smart watches which can measure pulse or even perform an EKG, can be helpful. If your patient is experiencing chest pain, you can have your patient palpate their chest to determine whether pain is reproducible. If there are significant cardiac concerns, refer your patient to the clinic or emergency department so they can be seen for an in-person evaluation.

Abdomen

Ask your patient if they are experiencing any stomach pain. You can have your patient palpate their abdomen themselves. See if they can localize the pain. Did you observe any guarding? Ask if the pain is worse when pressing on their abdomen or when letting go, such as in rebound tenderness. You could have them lay on a couch for this portion of the exam, especially if they are using a mobile device such as a phone or tablet. If a caregiver is also present, they may be able to help perform an abdominal exam or even assist in checking for costovertebral angle tenderness. Have your patient jump up and down. Did they experience any pain while jumping?

Extremities

Do you observe any swelling or color changes of your patient's extremities? Do you observe any clubbing of the fingertips?

Neurologic [54]

If there are significant neurologic concerns, have your patient be seen in person. You are able to perform some aspects virtually, however. Begin with performing a brief mental status exam. First, observe the patient's level of alertness. Then, test their orientation by asking them to state their name, their current location, and the time (year, month, day). Take note of any difficulty with speech, fast or slow speech, or confusion. Assess their attention by asking them to count down from 100 by 7 (serial sevens test) or to state the months of the year backward.

You can test some cranial nerve function virtually.

CN I Olfactory—ask your patient if they have any issues with their smell. This cranial nerve is rarely tested, even in person.

CN II Optic—Visual acuity cannot be accurately tested during a telemedicine visit, though you can ask your patient if they are experiencing blurry vision.

CN III Oculomotor, IV Trochlear, and VI Abducens—Have your patient look all the way to the left, right, up, and down to observe their extraocular movements. You may be able to observe nystagmus, as well as pupil symmetry.

CN V Trigeminal—You may ask the patient to check the sensation of their forehead, cheeks, and chin with their finger or facial tissue.

CN VII Facial—Have your patient raise their eyebrows, close their eyes tightly, smile, and puff out their cheeks.

CN VIII Vestibulocochlear—Hearing cannot be accurately tested during a telemedicine visit.

CN IX Glossopharyngeal, X Vagus—It is possible, though difficult, to observe your patient's palate elevation.

CN XI Spinal Accessory—Have your patient shrug their shoulders and look to the right and then the left.

CN XII Hypoglossal—You can have your patient stick out their tongue and then move their tongue from side to side.

You should be able to test gait, fine finger movements, rapid alternating movements, pronator drift, and active range of motion by coaching your patient through each step. However, it is not possible to accurately test reflexes or tone [54].

Case: Acute Sinusitis

You are a primary care pediatrician. You look at your schedule for this afternoon and see that you have a telemedicine visit with your patient, Jennifer, for nasal congestion. Jennifer is a 15-year-old with an unremarkable past medical history who you have known for the last 10 years. Your medical assistant meets with her first and reviews her medical and surgical history, allergies, and medications (there are no changes). Jennifer has a smartwatch which can measure her pulse and a thermometer, but she does not have a blood pressure cuff. The medical assistant has Jennifer check her pulse (86) and her temperature (37.2 °C).

Provider: *As Jennifer appears on screen, you observe her easy work of breathing and overall well appearance, though she looks a little tired. Her mom, Holly, is visible at the side of your screen.* Good to see you both. Jennifer, I'm sorry you're not feeling well.

Jennifer: Hi Doc.

Provider: Before we begin, I'd like to check a few things. First, can you see and hear me OK? I would also like to confirm a good phone number to reach you in case we get disconnected.

Jennifer: Yes, I can see and hear you. *Holly interjects with their home phone number. You then confirm her home address, which is in her electronic health record and accessible during the telemedicine visit.*

Provider: Thank you. Tell me what's been going on.

Jennifer: Well, about 3 weeks ago I had a cold. I had a fever for a couple days, and then a sore throat, runny nose, and cough. I haven't had a fever or a sore throat for a couple of weeks, but this runny nose won't go away. When I blow my nose, it's now dark yellow or brown. Last week, I went to the drug store near my house, and they tested me for COVID-19; it was negative.

Provider: For how long exactly have you been congested, and did the congestion ever go away entirely during that time?

Jennifer: I've been congested and blowing my nose every day for the past two and a half weeks. It's never gone away.

Provider: I see. Have you had any difficulty breathing? Have you still been able to keep yourself hydrated and have some things to eat?

Jennifer: I'm breathing fine. Yes, I've been able to eat and drink.

Provider: Have you taken anything to help with your symptoms?

Jennifer: I had been taking Tylenol or ibuprofen a couple of weeks ago, but I haven't taken any last week. I've been drinking tea with honey which has been really nice.

Provider: Have you ever tried using a neti pot or saline rinses for your nose? How about fluticasone nasal spray, which is a steroid spray that can help decrease inflammation in your nose.

Jennifer: My friend recommended using a neti pot, so I did try it out a couple times last week. It didn't really help. I haven't used any nasal sprays.

Provider: Are you experiencing any other symptoms? *You complete a full review of symptoms. She denies experiencing any other symptoms aside from rhinorrhea and nasal congestion.*

Provider: I'd now like to try and do a physical exam as best we can. Since we are meeting virtually today, I'll need your help. First, take your hands and feel along your neck. Is anything tender? Do you notice any lumps or bumps?

Now, please swallow. Was it painful to swallow? Did your ears pop when you swallowed?

I'd like to take a look in your nose and throat if I can. Holly, if you have your smartphone with you, can you shine the light into her mouth as she leans forward toward the camera? Then, can you shine the light into her nose as she leans forward again?

Now, press your fingers to your forehead. *You demonstrate how to check for sinus pain.* Now, can you please bend down with your head to the floor. Did you feel any increased pressure in your head?

Turn and look all the way to the right, and now all the way to the left. Now, drop your chin to your chest. Did you feel any neck tightness or stiffness?

While Jennifer is helping you with the physical exam, you observe that her eyes are clear without injection or icterus and her pupils are symmetric. Her breathing is comfortable. You don't hear any wheezing or see any nasal flaring or movement of her stomach, chest, or neck as she breathes. There are no rashes or lesions on her exposed skin.

She is not experiencing any pain or difficulty with swallowing. However, she is experiencing sinus pain and an increased feeling of pressure in her head, especially when she leaned forward. When you looked in her mouth, you saw non-erythematous normal-sized tonsils, but with some evidence of post-nasal drip. It was hard to see inside her nose due to video quality, but you could hear that she was congested, and she blew her nose throughout the visit. Her neck range of movement was full without stiffness.

Provider: Thank you for helping me with the physical exam. Based on the duration of your symptoms and your exam today, I think you have a sinus infection. What I'd like to have you do is use fluticasone, that nasal spray I mentioned before, twice a day for the next week to decrease the inflammation in your nose. Just prior to using the spray, use your neti pot. This will help clear your nasal passages. I'd like to set up a follow-up appointment with you in 1 week to check in on your symptoms. Often, we can treat sinus infections just with supportive care. But if you continue to have symptoms by our follow-up visit, we can also use antibiotics to clear the infection. What questions do you have for me?

Jennifer: That sounds good to me. How do I use the spray?

Holly: That sounds good. I'd like to avoid antibiotics if possible.

You demonstrate correct fluticasone spray technique. You enter a telemedicine appointment request in the electronic health record for 1 week from now.

Jennifer: Thanks, doc. See you next week. *Jennifer logs off.*

Other Topics in Primary Care of Adolescents

Reproductive, mental, substance use, eating disorders, and gender healthcare all come up within primary care practice, though have more detailed information elsewhere in this book. These concerns are discussed below from a primary care point of view. Please see their respective chapters for a more comprehensive look at each of these topics.

Reproductive Healthcare

Counseling for all types of contraception and providing combined oral contraceptives is feasible over telehealth [19]. There is precedent for starting such methods without a recent blood pressure measurement, with plans to check blood pressure at the next in-person visit [19]. Supplementation of telehealth visits with laboratory studies is required for pregnancy testing and STI screening, including routine HIV screening for patients on PrEP. Additionally, in some laboratories, it may be feasible to obtain self-swabs for yeast, trichomonas, and bacterial vaginosis, while this may otherwise require an in-person visit. In-person visits continue to be required for Papanicolaou smears, long-acting reversible contraceptive placement, medroxyprogesterone injections, and acute pelvic concerns [19]. Addressing dermatologic or other visible acute concerns in the breasts and genitourinary region remains a gray area within telemedicine at this time. Until best practice standards are introduced and accepted, providers must use their judgment to determine the best course of action, whether it be visualization over telemedicine, patient photographs uploaded to the electronic medical record through a patient portal, or requiring a follow-up in-person examination [19].

Mental Healthcare

Mental healthcare, including screening, diagnosis, and treatment, is an important part of primary care for adolescents. As discussed previously, it is recommended you incorporate standard screeners, such as the Patient Health Questionnaire-9 (PHQ-9), General Anxiety Disorder-7 (GAD-7), Screen for Child Anxiety Related Emotional Disorders (SCARED), or others that are used in your clinic. Most mental health concerns can be discussed thoroughly via telemedicine and often do not require an adjunct in-person visit or lab studies for diagnosis and treatment. However, patients will have varying preferences for discussing personal topics regarding mental health; while some patients may prefer the physical and emotional distance of telemedicine, others may prefer to discuss such personal concerns face-to-face [45]. It is important to elicit patient preference before and during such visits, considering changes to future appointments or the need to transition a virtual visit to in-person as needed.

Substance Use

Virtual visits for substance use disorders are limited in their reach by the current Drug Enforcement Agency guidelines and restrictions. This was expanded during COVID-19 to allow for providers to prescribe buprenorphine without an in-person visit, provided that the structured intake take place as required when funded by Substance Abuse and Mental Health Services Administration [19]. Providers should continue their typical substance use screening and counseling with primary care visits [55].

Disordered Eating

Accurate vitals and blind weights are required for outpatient monitoring of eating disorders [56]. These may be able to be accomplished by training caregivers at home. However, if this is not feasible, such visits may require an adjunct nurse visit or a local pediatrician visit or to be performed fully in person [19]. Electrolyte monitoring can be accomplished through laboratory visits as needed [19]. Privacy is important with all adolescent visits, but especially so with eating disorder care. Time and space for both patients and caregivers to have privacy with providers is important [19].

Gender Care

While provision of gender care may not typically fall into primary care, many gender-diverse patients will be seen for primary care, as well as to discuss referral for gender-affirming care as desired, and if not provided in the primary care setting. It is especially important to screen for mental health and safety for gender diverse patients, as they can experience higher rates of depression, suicidal ideation, and physical and sexual abuse [57]. As with all patients, screening and referral to appropriate resources should be performed, as gender-diverse teens experience further disenfranchisement in the form of housing insecurity, financial instability, or other limitations in social support when there is estrangement from caregivers, friends, or social/spiritual groups [57].

Limitations

Virtual care has many benefits for providers and families but is limited by several factors. These can be decreased by technology adjuncts for physical exams, photographs submitted for visible complaints, and supplemental visits, but they are not able to be eliminated. Deviations from the standard of care include complete vital sign measurements, vision screening, and physical exam (most commonly the heart, spine, and skin including indicators of self-harm or abuse in addition to rashes and lesions of concern, genital exams) [51].

It is unavoidable that some visits will require transition to an in-person visit. As noted previously, this can include need for testing, vaccinations, medication administration, and further physical examination. Visits should be transitioned if providers are unable to meet the standard of care for diagnosis and management of any patient concern [21, 58]. Visits may also need to be transitioned if technology is inadequate, such as poor Internet connection, poor video or audio quality, or significant delay in transmission [58]. Provider and patient comfort should also be considerations for transitioning visit type [58]. If patients are not acutely ill requiring immediate increase in the level of care, and if visit transition is not required due to technology malfunctions, you may offer the patient and family to continue with the visit and evaluate other concerns. This can limit the length of the in-person visit.

Vaccinations are an important component of well care that cannot be accomplished over telemedicine. In 2020, there was a significant decline in well visits. As would be expected with such a decrease, significant delays were seen in routine childhood vaccinations [18, 59, 60]. In the wake of high-infection phases of the pandemic, vaccine rates remain decreased from prior [18]. Influenza vaccination rates for the past 2 years have also significantly decreased from prior [61]. In order to provide timely catch-up vaccinations, as well as limit future ramifications for omitted vaccines or decreased herd immunity, it is imperative that appropriate in-person visits for vaccinations occur promptly in order to limit the potential for preventable disease outbreaks [18, 62]. No research is available regarding the percentage of teens accessing well visits via telemedicine who remain up to date with vaccinations. Vaccine counseling and adjunct nurse, public health department, or pharmacy visits to complete injections are vital.

Reimbursement

Reimbursement can be variable based on insurers and location of practice. Previously, poor reimbursement or coverage for virtual care was a significant barrier to embracing virtual care [63]. Starting in March 2020, a temporary waiver regarding regulations by the Health Insurance Portability and Accountability Act (HIPAA) was issued by the US government [63]. This allowed for rapid expansion of telemedicine, and it has provided for expanded use of technologies that may not, or have not, been shown to fully comply with HIPAA policy, as long as they are utilized by providers in good faith for the care of their patients [64]. This was most recently reaffirmed in January of 2021 [64]. It is recommended that workflows and software platforms migrate to HIPAA-compliant technology as soon as possible in order to protect patient privacy and ensure a seamless transition when this waiver expires [65]. Reimbursement is currently also variable across visit types and will likely continue to evolve over time.

Ending the Virtual Visit

In general, an abrupt ending should be avoided [12]. Discuss and confirm understanding of any plans made during the visit and schedule a follow-up appointment if needed. Always allow the patient to end the telemedicine visit first before leaving the visit yourself in case your patient has last-minute questions [1]. If staffing allows, consider developing a clinical workflow that allows medical assistant or scheduling to join the end of the visit to wrap up any final instructions and schedule the next appointment.

References

1. Health Resources and Services Administration. Conduct a telehealth physical exam 2022.
2. McConnochie KM, Wood NE, Kitzman HJ, Herendeen NE, Roy J, Roghmann KJ. Telemedicine reduces absence resulting from illness in urban child care: evaluation of an innovation. Pediatrics. 2005;115(5):1273–82.
3. McConnochie KM, Conners GP, Brayer AF, Goepp J, Herendeen NE, Wood NE, et al. Differences in diagnosis and treatment using telemedicine versus in-person evaluation of acute illness. Ambul Pediatr. 2006;6(4):187–95. discussion 96–7
4. Fleischman A, Hourigan SE, Lyon HN, Landry MG, Reynolds J, Steltz SK, et al. Creating an integrated care model for childhood obesity: a randomized pilot study utilizing telehealth in a community primary care setting. Clin Obes. 2016;6(6):380–8.
5. Ramaswamy A, Yu M, Drangsholt S, Ng E, Culligan PJ, Schlegel PN, et al. Patient satisfaction with telemedicine during the COVID-19 pandemic: retrospective cohort study. J Med Internet Res. 2020;22(9):e20786.
6. Halterman JS, Fagnano M, Tajon RS, Tremblay P, Wang H, Butz A, et al. Effect of the School-Based Telemedicine Enhanced Asthma Management (SB-TEAM) program on asthma morbidity: a randomized clinical trial. JAMA Pediatr. 2018;172(3):e174938.
7. Di Bartolo P, Nicolucci A, Cherubini V, Iafusco D, Scardapane M, Rossi MC. Young patients with type 1 diabetes poorly controlled and poorly compliant with self-monitoring of blood glucose: can technology help? Results of the i-NewTrend randomized clinical trial. Acta Diabetol. 2017;54(4):393–402.
8. Shah AC, Badawy SM. Telemedicine in pediatrics: systematic review of randomized controlled trials. JMIR Pediatr Parent. 2021;4(1):e22696.
9. Siew L, Hsiao A, McCarthy P, Agarwal A, Lee E, Chen L. Reliability of telemedicine in the assessment of seriously ill children. Pediatrics. 2016;137(3):e20150712.

10. Rokicki-Parashar J, Phadke A, Brown-Johnson C, Jee O, Sattler A, Torres E, et al. Transforming interprofessional roles during virtual health care: the evolving role of the medical assistant, in relationship to National Health Profession Competency Standards. J Prim Care Community Health. 2021;12:21501327211004285.
11. Gusdorf RE, Shah KP, Triana AJ, McCoy AB, Pabla B, Scoville E, et al. A patient education intervention improved rates of successful video visits during rapid implementation of telehealth. J Telemed Telecare. 2021;29:1357633X211008786.
12. Telehealth Etiquette: Good Screenside Manners for Successful Consults: Old Dominion University College of Health Sciences School of Nursing.
13. Rabatin AE, Lynch ME, Severson MC, Brandenburg JE, Driscoll SW. Pediatric telerehabilitation medicine: making your virtual visits efficient, effective and fun. J Pediatr Rehabil Med. 2020;13(3):355–70.
14. Alderman EM, Breuner CC, Committee on Adolescence. Unique needs of the adolescent. Pediatrics. 2019;144(6)
15. McNary A. Consent to treatment of minors. Innov Clin Neurosci. 2014;11(3–4):43–5.
16. Benziger CP, Huffman MD, Sweis RN, Stone NJ. The telehealth ten: a guide for a patient-assisted virtual physical examination. Am J Med. 2021;134(1):48–51.
17. Erkkola-Anttinen N, Irjala H, Laine MK, Tähtinen PA, Löyttyniemi E, Ruohola A. Smartphone otoscopy performed by parents. Telemed J E Health. 2019;25(6):477–84.
18. American Academy of Pediatrics. Guidance on providing pediatric well-care during COVID-19 2022.
19. Barney A, Buckelew S, Mesheriakova V, Raymond-Flesch M. The COVID-19 pandemic and rapid implementation of adolescent and young adult telemedicine: challenges and opportunities for innovation. J Adolesc Health. 2020;67(2):164–71.
20. Shim JY, Kaur R, Laufer MR, Grimstad FW. The use of telemedicine in pediatric and adolescent gynecology. J Pediatr Adolesc Gynecol. 2022;35(2):133–7.
21. Curfman A, Hackell JM, Herendeen NE, Alexander J, Marcin JP, Moskowitz WB, et al. Telehealth: opportunities to improve access, quality, and cost in pediatric care. Pediatrics. 2022;149(3):e2021056035.
22. Gilkey MB, Kong WY, Huang Q, Grabert BK, Thompson P, Brewer NT. Using telehealth to deliver primary care to adolescents during and after the COVID-19 pandemic: National Survey Study of US Primary Care Professionals. J Med Internet Res. 2021;23(9):e31240.
23. Spitzer RL, Kroenke K, Williams JB, Löwe B. A brief measure for assessing generalized anxiety disorder: the GAD-7. Arch Intern Med. 2006;166(10):1092–7.
24. Kroenke K, Spitzer RL, Williams JB. The PHQ-9: validity of a brief depression severity measure. J Gen Intern Med. 2001;16(9):606–13.
25. Peddecord KM, Wang W, Wang L, Ralston K, Ly E, Friedman L, et al. Adolescents' self-reported recall of anticipatory guidance provided during well-visits at nine medical clinics in San Diego, California, 2009–2011. J Adolesc Health. 2016;58(3):267–75.
26. Richardson L, Parker EO, Zhou C, Kientz J, Ozer E, McCarty C. Electronic health risk behavior screening with integrated feedback among adolescents in primary care: randomized controlled trial. J Med Internet Res. 2021;23(3):e24135.
27. Pooni R, Pageler NM, Sandborg C, Lee T. Pediatric subspecialty telemedicine use from the patient and provider perspective. Pediatr Res. 2022;91(1):241–6.
28. Legano LA, Desch LW, Messner SA, Idzerda S, Flaherty EG, COCAA NEGLECT, Council on Children with Disabilities, et al. Maltreatment of children with disabilities. Pediatrics. 2021;147(5):e2021050920.
29. Flynn JT, Kaelber DC, Baker-Smith CM, Blowey D, Carroll AE, Daniels SR, et al. Clinical practice guideline for screening and management of high blood pressure in children and adolescents. Pediatrics. 2017;140(3):e20171904.
30. Campisi SC, Marchand JD, Siddiqui FJ, Islam M, Bhutta ZA, Palmert MR. Can we rely on adolescents to self-assess puberty stage? A systematic review and meta-analysis. J Clin Endocrinol Metab. 2020;105(8):2846.

31. Peng X, Peng Y, Li Y, Nie X, Gong C, Wu D, et al. Validity of web-based self-assessment of pubertal development against pediatrician assessments. Pediatr Investig. 2018;2(3):141–8.
32. Hunt WR, Linnemann RW, Middour-Oxler B. Transition planning for chronic illnesses in the time of COVID-19. J Patient Exp. 2020;7(6):848–50.
33. White PH, Cooley WC, Group TCRA, Pediatrics AAO, Physicians AAOF, Physicians ACO. Supporting the health care transition from adolescence to adulthood in the medical home. Pediatrics. 2018;142(5):e20182587.
34. Cahan EM, Mittal V, Shah NR, Thadaney-Israni S. Achieving a quintuple aim for telehealth in pediatrics. Pediatr Clin N Am. 2020;67(4):683–705.
35. Patel ML, Wakayama LN, Bass MB, Breland JY. Motivational interviewing in eHealth and telehealth interventions for weight loss: a systematic review. Prev Med. 2019;126:105738.
36. Matheson EM, King DE, Everett CJ. Healthy lifestyle habits and mortality in overweight and obese individuals. J Am Board Fam Med. 2012;25(1):9–15.
37. Martinez M, Kanter D, Turk M. Health and wellness for children with disabilities. In: Kliegman R, Stanton B, Behrman R, St. Geme J, Schor N, editors. Nelson textbook of Pediatrics. 20th ed. Philadelphia: Elsevier; 2020. p. e3769–73.
38. Houtrow A, Elias ER, Davis BE, Disabilities COCW. Promoting healthy sexuality for children and adolescents with disabilities. Pediatrics. 2021;148(1):e2021052043.
39. Shingleton RM, Palfai TP. Technology-delivered adaptations of motivational interviewing for health-related behaviors: a systematic review of the current research. Patient Educ Couns. 2016;99(1):17–35.
40. Döbler A, Herbeck Belnap B, Pollmann H, Farin E, Raspe H, Mittag O. Telephone-delivered lifestyle support with action planning and motivational interviewing techniques to improve rehabilitation outcomes. Rehabil Psychol. 2018;63(2):170–81.
41. Stevens J, Hayes J, Pakalnis A. A randomized trial of telephone-based motivational interviewing for adolescent chronic headache with medication overuse. Cephalalgia. 2014;34(6):446–54.
42. Hides L, Quinn C, Chan G, Cotton S, Pocuca N, Connor JP, et al. Telephone-based motivational interviewing enhanced with individualised personality-specific coping skills training for young people with alcohol-related injuries and illnesses accessing emergency or rest/recovery services: a randomized controlled trial (QuikFix). Addiction. 2021;116(3):474–84.
43. Constant HMRM, Ferigolo M, Barros HMT, Moret-Tatay C. A clinical trial on a brief motivational intervention in reducing alcohol consumption under a telehealth supportive counseling. Psychiatry Res. 2021;303:114068.
44. Chandler AL, Beavers JC, Hall RW. Telemedicine in pediatrics: possibilities and pitfalls. Pediatr Rev. 2020;41(7):376–8.
45. Hawke LD, Sheikhan NY, MacCon K, Henderson J. Going virtual: youth attitudes toward and experiences of virtual mental health and substance use services during the COVID-19 pandemic. BMC Health Serv Res. 2021;21(1):340.
46. Sinsky CA, Jerzak JT, Hopkins KD. Telemedicine and team-based care: the perils and the promise. Mayo Clin Proc. 2021;96(2):429–37.
47. Fletcher SE, Tsang VWL. The era of virtual care: perspectives of youth on virtual appointments in COVID-19 and beyond. Paediatr Child Health. 2021;26(4):210–3.
48. Kemery DC, Goldschmidt K. Can you see me? Can you hear me? Best practices for videoconference-enhanced telemedicine visits for children. J Pediatr Nurs. 2020;55:261–3.
49. Myers K, Nelson EL, Rabinowitz T, Hilty D, Baker D, Barnwell SS, et al. American telemedicine association practice guidelines for telemental health with children and adolescents. Telemed J E Health. 2017;23(10):779–804.
50. Wood SM, Pickel J, Phillips AW, Baber K, Chuo J, Maleki P, et al. Acceptability, feasibility, and quality of telehealth for adolescent health care delivery during the COVID-19 pandemic: cross-sectional study of patient and family experiences. JMIR Pediatr Parent. 2021;4(4):e32708.
51. Wenderlich A, Herendeen N. Telehealth in pediatric primary care. Curr Probl Pediatr Adolesc Health Care. 2021;51:100951.

52. Wilson E, Free C, Morris TP, Syred J, Ahamed I, Menon-Johansson AS, et al. Internet-accessed sexually transmitted infection (e-STI) testing and results service: a randomised, single-blind, controlled trial. PLoS Med. 2017;14(12):e1002479.
53. Simon MA. Responding to intimate partner violence during telehealth clinical encounters. JAMA. 2021;325(22):2307–8.
54. Al Hussona M, Maher M, Chan D, Micieli JA, Jain JD, Khosravani H, et al. The virtual neurologic exam: instructional videos and guidance for the COVID-19 era. Can J Neurol Sci. 2020;47(5):598–603.
55. Morin KA, Parrotta MD, Eibl JK, Marsh DC. A retrospective cohort study comparing in-person and telemedicine-based opioid agonist treatment in Ontario, Canada, using administrative health data. Eur Addict Res. 2021;27(4):268–76.
56. Hornberger LL, Lane MA, Committee on Adolescence. Identification and management of eating disorders in children and adolescents. Pediatrics. 2021;147(1):e2020040279.
57. Newcomb ME, Hill R, Buehler K, Ryan DT, Whitton SW, Mustanski B. High burden of mental health problems, substance use, violence, and related psychosocial factors in transgender, non-binary, and gender diverse youth and young adults. Arch Sex Behav. 2020;49(2):645–59.
58. McSwain SD, Bernard J, Burke BL, Cole SL, Dharmar M, Hall-Barrow J, et al. American telemedicine association operating procedures for pediatric telehealth. Telemed J E Health. 2017;23(9):699–706.
59. Chandir S, Siddiqi DA. Inequalities in COVID-19 disruption of routine immunisations and returning to pre-COVID immunisation rates. Lancet Reg Health West Pac. 2021;10:100156.
60. Ota MOC, Badur S, Romano-Mazzotti L, Friedland LR. Impact of COVID-19 pandemic on routine immunization. Ann Med. 2021;53(1):2286–97.
61. Centers for Disease Control and Prevention. Influenza. National Center for Health Statistics 2022.
62. Dinleyici EC, Borrow R, Safadi MAP, van Damme P, Munoz FM. Vaccines and routine immunization strategies during the COVID-19 pandemic. Hum Vaccin Immunother. 2021;17(2):400–7.
63. Badawy SM, Radovic A. Digital approaches to remote pediatric health care delivery during the COVID-19 pandemic: existing evidence and a call for further research. JMIR Pediatr Parent. 2020;3(1):e20049.
64. Office for Civil Rights. Notification of enforcement discretion for telehealth remote communications during the COVID-19 Nationwide Public Health Emergency: U.S. Department of Health and Human Services; 2021.
65. Allgaier K, Schmid J, Hollmann K, Reusch PA, Conzelmann A, Renner TJ. Times are changing: digitalisation in child and adolescent psychotherapy. Eur Child Adolesc Psychiatry. 2021;30(11):1667–70.

Chapter 7
Sexual and Reproductive Health

Amanda E. Bryson, Florencia D. Kantt, Amy D. DiVasta, and Sarah Pitts

Background

The use of telemedicine for adolescent sexual and reproductive health services was widely and rapidly implemented at the onset of the COVID-19 pandemic to maintain continuity in sexual and reproductive healthcare while limiting in-person contact [1–6]. Prior to the COVID-19 pandemic, telemedicine services for sexual and reproductive healthcare were limited. However, mobile phone applications, messaging services, telephone calls, and live audiovisual communication had been previously utilized in the USA and globally to provide family planning services [7]. Such interventions were found to increase contraceptive method continuation and improve contraception knowledge, as well as being appropriate for determining contraception eligibility [7]. Given the relatively recent adaptation of widespread telemedicine services for sexual and reproductive healthcare, there is a paucity of literature examining its use and outcomes, especially within the adolescent population. The aim of this chapter is to provide the reader with practical guidance, informed by the available literature, to aid in the clinical use of telemedicine for adolescent sexual and reproductive health services, as this modality could serve as an important tool for such care beyond the pandemic [3–5, 8].

Amy D. DiVasta and Sarah Pitts are co-senior authors.

A. E. Bryson (✉) · F. D. Kantt · A. D. DiVasta · S. Pitts
Division of Adolescent & Young Adult Medicine, Boston Children's Hospital,
Boston, MA, USA
e-mail: Amanda.Bryson@childrens.harvard.edu; Amy.DiVasta@childrens.harvard.edu;
Sarah.Pitts@childrens.harvard.edu

© The Author(s), under exclusive license to Springer Nature
Switzerland AG 2024
Y. N. Evans et al. (eds.), *Telemedicine for Adolescent and Young Adult Health Care*, https://doi.org/10.1007/978-3-031-55760-6_7

We will focus on the use of synchronous telemedicine services for adolescent sexual and reproductive healthcare via either virtual or telephone visits, which will be referred to broadly as telemedicine throughout this chapter. Synchronous telemedicine requires bidirectional communication between a patient and a healthcare professional in real time [9]. A virtual visit includes two-way audio and video communication between a clinician and a patient, whereas a telephone visit would allow for audio communication only [9]. The use of other telehealth modalities (i.e., mobile phone applications or messaging services) is beyond the scope of this chapter.

Acceptability

While telemedicine for sexual and reproductive healthcare has advantages and disadvantages (Table 7.1), this modality is acceptable to clinicians and patients. Recent research found that clinicians providing telemedicine contraceptive services and adults utilizing telemedicine for contraceptive counseling were satisfied with these visits (80% of clinicians; 86% of patients), and respondents agree that telemedicine for contraceptive counseling should continue (84% of clinicians; 72% of patients) beyond the COVID-19 pandemic [10, 11]. In another survey, roughly one-third (39%) of US primary care providers included had used telemedicine for adolescent sexual health visits and contraceptive counseling [12]. Importantly, most of these providers thought that telemedicine increased adolescent access to care (69%) and supported continued use (67%) and reimbursement (92%) of telemedicine services [12].

Table 7.1 Advantages and disadvantages for adolescents using sexual and reproductive health telemedicine services [2, 3, 5, 6, 12, 13]

Advantages	Disadvantages
• Preventing exposure to infectious disease • Putting family at ease • Reducing transportation, time, and burden • Increasing access to care[a] • Meeting the adolescent where they are • Increasing continuity of care with medical home	• Inability to perform vital signs, certain examinations, and laboratory testing • Inability to deliver care across state lines[b] • Technology issues/availability • Lack of privacy/confidentiality • Inability to provide all contraceptive methods during the visit (i.e., LARC)

[a] Use of telemedicine can increase access for certain populations, like people living in rural communities. Gaps in telemedicine care continue to exist due to systemic inequities. Intentional interventions are needed to ensure equitable access to telemedicine access all populations
[b] Depends on a state's requirements for the provider to hold a license in the state where the patient is located

Fig. 7.1 Tips and tricks for a successful telemedicine visit for adolescent reproductive and sexual healthcare

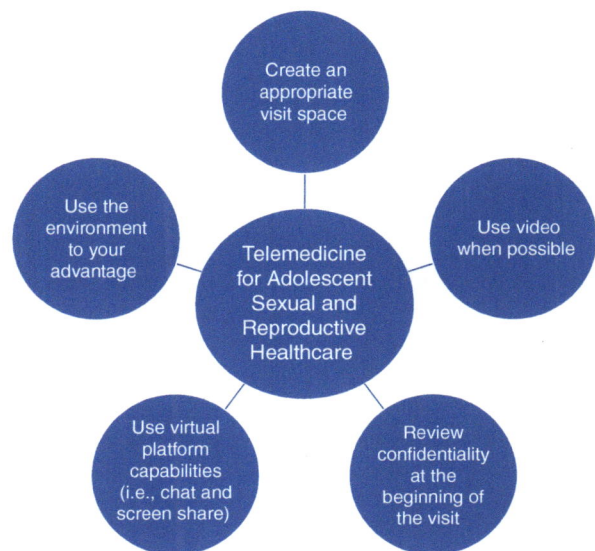

While research in this area is limited, the patient-clinician relationship can be formed during telemedicine visits, especially when using synchronous modalities with real-time audio and video capabilities to allow for the exchange of verbal and nonverbal cues [2, 13]. Establishing rapport with the patient and creating a welcoming space for adolescents during sexual and reproductive health telemedicine visits is key, given the personal and sensitive information discussed during these healthcare encounters.

We recommend the following "tips and tricks" (Fig. 7.1) to optimize telemedicine visits for adolescent sexual and reproductive healthcare. The provider should establish a quiet and professional environment in which to conduct telemedicine visits [2]. Whenever possible, the provider should have their video on to allow for nonverbal communication to cultivate the patient-clinician relationship [2, 13]. The provider should review confidentiality at the beginning of the visit and ensure the adolescent is in a space where they can have confidential conversations about their sexual and reproductive health (see Chap. 2 on confidentiality) [5, 14]. We recommend providers become familiar with the capabilities of their virtual visit platforms. Providers can enhance telemedicine visits by using the chat function to share information with patients (e.g., links to websites) or using the screen sharing function to provide patient education (e.g., contraceptive decision aid tools). Lastly, providers can use their environment to their advantage. For instance, if an adolescent is presenting with breakthrough bleeding while taking a combined oral contraceptive pill (cOCP), the provider can ask the adolescent if they have access to their pill pack. The provider can visualize the pill pack to determine if any pills have been missed and review how to appropriately take the medication.

Health Equity, Structural Racism, and Reproductive Justice

Disparities in sexual and reproductive healthcare are well documented. These disparities occur as a result of multiple intersecting systemic oppressions and threaten a person's reproductive autonomy [15]. Some of the current disparities in the USA include (1) increased barriers to non-coercive and comprehensive contraceptive care for people with low income, persons of color, transgender/gender diverse individuals, people who are incarcerated or detained, and people with disabilities; (2) reduced access to general reproductive healthcare for immigrant and Latinx populations; and (3) limited access to abortion services based on insurance status, immigration status, socioeconomic class, age, and zip code [16].

Reproductive justice is a contemporary reproductive rights and social justice framework created by Black women illustrating that the experience of reproduction is influenced by various intersecting factors such as race/ethnicity, class, immigration status, gender identity, sexuality, incarceration, ability, and religion [15]. Reproductive justice centers the following human rights: (1) the right not to have a child, (2) the right to have a child, (3) the right to parent children in safe and healthy environments, and (4) the right to maintain personal bodily autonomy, sexual autonomy, and gender freedom [15]. The reproductive justice framework derives its vital depth from drawing attention to the persistence of historical oppression and the ways in which white supremacy and capitalism can affect an individual's experience with reproduction, particularly for Black, Indigenous, and people of color, who have been (and continue to be) intentionally targeted throughout US history [15]. Guided by the tenets of reproductive justice, clinicians caring for adolescents can play a central role in mitigating barriers for adolescents seeking reproductive health services to improve health outcomes [16].

It is important to recognize that current disparities in and barriers to sexual and reproductive healthcare have been exacerbated in the context of the COVID-19 pandemic, especially for those in historically excluded communities. Such disparities could be amplified through use of telemedicine services. Telemedicine is an effective tool to expand access to care. However, its reliance on new technologies predictably uncovered and occasionally worsened disparities in access to the digital world, particularly for patients from families with fewer technological resources or poorer health literacy who would benefit most from expanded access through ongoing telemedicine-enabled healthcare (see Chap. 3 on equity) [17].

Inequities and disparities in telemedicine access, uptake, and visit completion are well documented in the research conducted prior to the COVID-19 pandemic. While data specific to disparities in telemedicine for reproductive health services are limited, previous findings suggest potential differences in the use of telemedicine for family planning services during the onset of the COVID-19 pandemic response—particularly in Black/African American and multiracial patients, who were less likely to use telemedicine services compared to in-person care [18]. Inequities can also be worsened by insurance, facility, or clinician-specific policies that require video contact during a telemedicine visit. Adolescents from families with low income may be less likely to have access to a suitable private physical space from which to participate in an audio-video telemedicine encounter. This presents unique challenges in the setting of adolescent reproductive healthcare, where protecting privacy and confidentiality is an integral component of high-quality care [14].

Despite its limitations, telemedicine can effectively bridge the service gap for the delivery of healthcare, provided that principles for achieving health equity are used in its planning and delivery. Efforts to address existing barriers to telemedicine uptake among historically excluded populations require an approach that acknowledges the impact of systemic racism and discrimination in medicine while simultaneously implementing and advocating for strategies to improve trust and digital literacy and expand access to reliable technology [19]. Equitable, patient-centered implementation of telemedicine family planning services thus requires a collective effort, centering the reproductive justice framework, to eliminate barriers and optimize widespread access to high-quality reproductive healthcare for all adolescents.

Sexual Health Counseling and Sexually Transmitted Infections

Sexual and reproductive health services are critical aspects of adolescent health [14]. The Society for Adolescent Health and Medicine endorses the exploration of alternative strategies, in addition to clinic encounters, to ensure all adolescents have access to sexual and reproductive services [14]. Telemedicine encounters may play an important role in increasing access to sexual and reproductive health services, including their use for general counseling and sexually transmitted infection (STI) screening and treatment [8, 9].

NM is a 15-year-old who presents via *telemedicine for a routine health maintenance exam. During the social history, NM reports they recently became sexually active.*

Counseling

Telemedicine encounters can be used to counsel adolescents on healthy sexual behaviors [8, 9]. Providers can perform routinely recommended sexual health screening and education, such as asking adolescents about sexual partners and practices, counseling on healthy relationships and sexual consent, and screening for teen dating violence via telemedicine [9, 14]. Prior to screening for dating violence, the provider must ensure the adolescent is in a confidential and safe place (see Chap. 2 on confidentiality). It is important for the provider to recognize screening for dating violence during a telemedicine visit could put the adolescent at risk [20]. The adolescent should help determine whether or not dating violence is discussed and, if so, in what manner it is discussed during a telemedicine encounter. If indicated, the provider can share dating violence resources (i.e., websites and hotlines) and perform safety planning using the screen sharing or chat function (https://www.loveis-respect.org/personal-safety/create-a-safety-plan/).

Providers can assess for desire for contraception and discuss strategies to reduce STI acquisition via telemedicine. When discussing barrier method use, it is important to recognize that many adolescents rely on in-person visits to obtain these methods, which would be impacted by telemedicine care [21]. Therefore, providers should use creative ways to ensure adolescents have access to barrier methods, such as ordering condoms by mail (search "free condoms by mail" plus the adolescent's location), directing patients to locations in the community providing free condoms and lubricant (https://condomfinder.org/#find-condoms), or arranging for a barrier method pickup appointment in the clinic. Providers can perform a human immunodeficiency virus (HIV) risk assessment and discuss pre-exposure prophylaxis (PrEP) [9]. If an adolescent is interested in PrEP, the provider can counsel the patient on the indications for and use of PrEP. Following counseling, the patient could attend an asynchronous lab visit prior to PrEP initiation. An in-person visit would be required if the adolescent chooses to receive PrEP via intramuscular (IM) injection (cabotegravir), which was approved by the US Food and Drug Administration (FDA) in December 2021 [22].

Routine screening for STIs among adolescents is widely recommended given the disproportionate rates of STIs in this age group [23]. Despite these recommendations, only one-fifth of sexually active US high school students report being screened for STIs [23]. Adolescents experience barriers to STI testing, including concerns about confidentiality, stigma, limited knowledge about sexual health, cost, and transportation to clinic [23]. Given these barriers, it is important to ensure that routine screening for STIs does not decline as a result of increased telemedicine utilization. STI screening should be performed based on guidelines that are informed by regional epidemiology [14]. Providers can discuss indication for screening and pursue asynchronous testing (i.e., a telemedicine visit followed by a lab visit) or home testing [24].

NM is interested in routine STI screening. NM chooses to schedule an asynchronous lab visit to perform the testing. NM's urine sample returns with a positive result for Chlamydia trachomatis. The provider calls NM to disclose the result and NM requests a telemedicine visit to discuss the result and treatment options in more detail.

Sexually Transmitted Infections (STIs)

Adolescents may prefer to receive treatment for STIs via telemedicine. The Centers for Disease Control and Prevention (CDC) recommends directly observed therapy (DOT) for either the first dose of a 7-day regimen (i.e., doxycycline 100 mg twice per day or levofloxacin 500 mg once per day) or the entirety of a single dose regimen (i.e., azithromycin 1 g) for the treatment of *Chlamydia trachomatis* [25]. However, with the shift toward use of 7-day regimens as first-line therapy, per updated CDC guidelines, [25] and an increase in telemedicine, providers and patients may wish to use pharmacy prescriptions for treatment in lieu of DOT [26]. One study showed that pharmacy prescriptions for *Chlamydia* treatment were used in roughly 60% of cases (n = 199) without significant delays in time to treatment (1.5 days for DOT vs. 3 days for prescriptions; $p = 0.08$) [26]. Therefore, if in line with patient preferences, it is reasonable to use telemedicine to treat *Chlamydia trachomatis* and *Trichomonas vaginalis* with oral medication regimens. An in-person visit is recommended for any patient with symptoms of pelvic inflammatory disease, at risk for complications, [3] requiring a genital exam or speculum exam, in need of IM treatment (*Neisseria gonorrhea* or syphilis), or by their preference. Treatment can be offered empirically after a known exposure or for a confirmed infection from laboratory testing. If a patient receives treatment via telemedicine, the provider should discuss the need for additional STI testing with the adolescent. The provider should also assist in arranging for a test of cure in 1 month for pregnant adolescents or test of reinfection in 3 months for non-pregnant adolescents [25]. Lastly, the provider should discuss partner notification and treatment, including expedited partner therapy, as permitted by law [25].

NM presents for a follow-up telemedicine visit. The provider assesses for signs and symptoms of a Chlamydia infection. NM is asymptomatic. The provider discusses disclosure of infection to sexual partners and treatment options. The provider prescribes doxycycline 100 mg twice per day for 7 days. The provider arranges for additional STI testing and reviews strategies to reduce STI acquisition.

Vulvovaginitis

Vulvovaginitis, inflammation of the vulva and vagina, is one of the most common gynecologic concerns [27]. Therefore, understanding appropriate use of telemedicine for evaluation and treatment of vulvovaginitis is important. In addition to patient preference for in-person evaluation, adolescents with signs/symptoms of pelvic inflammatory disease (i.e., fever, abdominal/pelvic pain, post-coital bleeding, abnormal uterine bleeding (AUB), mucopurulent discharge) or recurrent symptoms should be triaged to in-person evaluation.

Few studies have evaluated the use of telemedicine for vulvovaginal concerns. In one report of telemedicine visits for 12 pediatric and adolescent patients presenting with vulvovaginal complaints, one-third of patients required a follow-up in-person visit within the 90 days of the telemedicine encounter [28]. While follow-up evaluations to ensure resolution of symptoms were not performed, these preliminary findings suggest that two-thirds of the patients were adequately treated via telemedicine. While evidence guiding the use of telemedicine for vulvovaginal concerns is lacking, expert consensus suggests that empiric treatment for bacterial vaginosis, vulvovaginal candidiasis, and trichomoniasis is generally benign and in-person follow-up should be recommended if there is inadequate treatment response [24].

Vulvovaginitis Evaluation

While telemedicine limits vulvovaginal evaluation given the inability to perform an external genital exam, speculum exam, and/or testing (e.g., vaginal pH, amine test, wet preparation with microscopy, laboratory testing), knowledge of epidemiology and a thorough history can help guide management. While most vaginal discharge is physiologic, the most common causes of adolescent vulvovaginitis are bacterial vaginosis, vulvovaginal candidiasis, and trichomoniasis [27]. The medical history should include onset and duration of symptoms, association of symptoms with sexual activity or menstruation, description of vaginal discharge (i.e., color, consistency, quantity, odor), other associated symptoms (e.g., pruritus, pain, skin irritation, dysuria, dyspareunia), medication history (e.g., hormonal contraceptives, antibiotics, and steroids), medical history (e.g., diabetes, immunosuppression), use of vulvovaginal products (e.g., douches, soaps, lubricants, or other products), and sexual history [27]. Based on this history, the provider can use their best clinical judgement to determine whether the discharge is physiologic or pathologic.

Physiologic Vaginal Discharge

Physiologic discharge is likely in the absence of odor, pruritus, pain, dysuria, or vulvovaginal irritation [27]. If physiologic discharge is suspected based on history during a telemedicine encounter, the provider should educate the adolescent about normal vaginal discharge, factors that can change vaginal discharge consistency and quantity (e.g., menstruation, hormonal contraceptives, pregnancy), and factors that increase the risk of vulvovaginitis (e.g., use of douches and other vulvovaginal products, exposure to sexually transmitted infections) [27]. It is important to avoid treatment of physiologic discharge, as unnecessary antibiotic courses can disrupt the vaginal microbiome. An in-person follow-up visit can be scheduled if the adolescent remains concerned about vaginal discharge for further evaluation and education.

If physiologic discharge is suspected during a telemedicine visit, the clinicians should use this opportunity to empower the adolescent with information about normal vaginal discharge. This knowledge may help mitigate feelings of shame about vaginal hygiene and reduce the likelihood of using products marketed to improve vaginal hygiene which can lead to abnormal vaginal discharge and other complications. Intravaginal practices, such as wiping, cleansing, or douching, are influenced by various complex social, cultural, environmental, and biological factors. Clinicians should be aware that adolescents' intravaginal practices and motivations for these practices differ across racial and ethnic groups, and beliefs regarding vulvovaginal hygiene practices are heavily influenced by social and cultural norms [29, 30]. Understanding adolescent's perspectives on vaginal health, including the strong trans-generational nature of intravaginal practices particularly in Black and Latinx adolescents, and knowing their vaginal hygiene practices can help clinicians develop effective counseling messages, anticipatory guidance, and tailored interventions to support adolescents in achieving optimal vulvovaginal health [31, 32].

Infectious Vulvovaginitis

While many people with bacterial vaginosis are asymptomatic, it is the most common cause of abnormal vaginal discharge among adolescents [27]. Bacterial vaginosis is caused by overgrowth of anaerobic bacteria (i.e., *Gardnerella vaginalis, Prevotella, Mobiluncus, Ureaplasma, and Mycoplasma*) and reduction of *lactobacilli* [27]. The discharge is classically described as thin, white-gray, and homogenous discharge with a fishy odor. The odor may be more noticeable after sex [27]. Risk factors for developing bacterial vaginosis include sexual activity and practices (e.g., new partners, lack of condom use), use of douches or other vulvovaginal products, and chronic stress [27]. Adolescents reporting discharge consistent with bacterial vaginosis, especially in the setting of risk factors, could be treated empirically with oral or intravaginal metronidazole or intravaginal clindamycin via a telemedicine encounter and should be counseled to follow-up in-person if symptoms worsen, persist, or recur [24]. Additionally, as the presence of bacterial vaginosis can increase the risk of STI acquisition, STI testing should be discussed with the patient [27].

Vulvovaginal candidiasis is caused by the presence of vaginal yeast, most commonly *Candida albicans* [27]. The vaginal discharge is often described as thick, white, and curd-like and is associated with vulvar pruritus and irritation. In the absence of a co-occurring infection, the discharge is typically odorless [27]. Adolescents who are immunocompromised, living with HIV, diagnosed with diabetes mellitus, and/or are pregnant are at higher risk of *Candida* overgrowth. Certain medications, such as steroids and recent antibiotic use, also increase risk of vulvovaginal candidiasis [27]. Adolescents with a clinical history suggesting uncomplicated vulvovaginal candidiasis can be treated empirically with over-the-counter intravaginal azoles or oral fluconazole via a telemedicine encounter and should be counseled to follow-up in-person should symptoms worsen, persist, or recur [24, 27].

Trichomoniasis is caused by infection with the protozoan *Trichomoniasis vaginalis*, the most prevalent nonviral STI in the USA [27]. The discharge is typically described as copious, yellow-green, frothy, and malodorous. While many adolescents with *T. vaginalis* infections are asymptomatic, other common symptoms are vulvar irritation, pruritus, dysuria, dyspareunia, and post-coital bleeding [27]. Adolescents who are sexually active, do not use barrier methods, and douche are at increased risk of acquiring *T. vaginalis*. Adolescents reporting discharge and symptoms consistent with trichomoniasis, especially in the setting of risk factors, can be treated empirically with oral metronidazole via a telemedicine encounter and should be counseled to follow-up in-person should symptoms worsen, persist, or recur [24]. Additionally, comprehensive STI testing should be discussed with the patient. Lastly, expedited partner therapy for trichomoniasis should be discussed as is allowable by law [27].

Contraception and Menstrual Management

Telemedicine can be used to provide many contraceptive services safely and effectively, including counseling, initiation, surveillance, and side effect management (Table 7.2) [1, 3, 4, 8, 33, 34]. Provision of contraceptive services via telemedicine may play an important role in expanding access to those who face barriers to in-person care [35]. Telemedicine can also be used to evaluate/manage menstrual disorders and for menstrual suppression [24, 28, 36].

AG is a 15-year-old adolescent who calls to make an appointment to discuss contraception. AG reports it is difficult for them to come to clinic and is wondering if the visit can be virtual. The administrator asks if AG knows what type of contraception they would like. AG is not sure yet. The administrator schedules AG for a telemedicine contraceptive counseling visit.

Table 7.2 Indications for contraceptive services via telemedicine

	POPs	CHC	DMPA	Implant	IUD
Counseling	Y	Y	Y	Y	Y
Method initiation	Y	Y (if normal BP within 12 months)	DMPA-SC: Y	N	N
			DMPA-IM: N		
Surveillance[a]	Y	Y	Y	Y	Y
Switching or discontinuing method[b]	Y	Y	Y	N	N

POP progesterone-only pills, *CHC* combined hormonal contraception, *DMPA* depot medroxyprogesterone acetate, *IUD* intrauterine device, *SC* subcutaneous, *IM* intramuscular, *Y* yes, *N*, no
[a] Except if heavy bleeding, severe pelvic pain, or concern for ectopic pregnancy (all methods), nonpalpable device (implant), or concern for missing strings, device expulsion, or pregnancy (IUD)
[b] Switching to non-LARC method

Contraceptive Counseling

There is a wide support for contraceptive counseling via telemedicine [1, 3, 4, 8, 9, 37]. As per best practices, counseling should be patient-centered, comprehensive, and nondirective [38]. Key components of patient-centered contraceptive counseling include reviewing past contraception history and experiences, asking about patient preferences, identifying contraindications to methods, sharing knowledge about medically appropriate options, exploring obstacles to decision-making, and assessing the patient's desire to start the method immediately, [20, 38, 39] all of which can be accomplished virtually. Providers can refer to the CDC US Medical Eligibility Criteria (MEC) for Contraceptive Use 2016 guidelines to assess for method contraindications (access available via the Internet or mobile phone applications) [40]. Providers can utilize the screen-sharing function of a video visit platform to review a contraceptive decision aid (such as https://picck.org/resource/curated-contraception-decision-aids/) to enhance counseling during a telemedicine visit [20].

If the patient wishes to start contraception immediately, many contraceptive methods can be started on the same day as the telemedicine visit for contraceptive counseling. Exceptions to the "quick start" via telemedicine visits include the contraceptive implant, intrauterine devices (IUDs), depot medroxyprogesterone acetate via IM injection (DMPA-IM), and diaphragms requiring in-office fitting. While actual placement of long-acting reversible contraception (LARC) methods cannot be achieved via telemedicine, a virtual visit can be useful for LARC counseling [4]. Such counseling could include review of indications for use, efficacy, potential contraindications, expected bleeding profile and side effects, alternative methods, and what to expect during the insertion procedure [4]. Access to accurate LARC counseling is limited in the USA and globally and is influenced by provider and clinic characteristics [41]. Therefore, some adolescents may need to seek subspecialty care for LARC services. The use of telemedicine visits for LARC-specific counseling may help to increase adolescent access to LARC services by decreasing barriers associated with in-person care, such as transportation, time, and cost. However, it is imperative that the use of telemedicine services for LARC counseling does not create barriers for adolescents, such as impeding same day LARC provision. Ultimately, telemedicine for LARC counseling should be utilized for adolescents who remain undecided about whether they desire LARC and who want more information about options. If the adolescent desires LARC placement following virtual contraceptive counseling, the provider can offer a contraceptive bridge method while the patient waits for their LARC insertion [8, 20]. An additional in-person visit prior to LARC insertion is not required, as the evidence does not support need for examination, STI testing, or measurement of body mass index (BMI) prior to the insertion visit [42].

At the telemedicine contraceptive counseling visit, AG reports that their first sexual encounter was 1 month ago. AG is interested in starting a contraceptive method to help prevent pregnancy in addition to condoms. AG has never used hormonal contraception before. AG would like a method that is effective at preventing pregnancy but doesn't want any method that requires a procedure. AG does not have any chronic medical conditions and is not currently taking any medications. The provider determines AG is eligible for all contraceptive methods and shares their screen to review a contraceptive decision aid together. Based on this discussion, AG would like to start combined oral contraceptive pills (cOCPs). AG is confident about being able to take the pill every day. AG asks if they can start the pills today.

Contraceptive Initiation

Contraceptive provision via telemedicine has been widely endorsed [1, 3, 4, 9, 33, 34]. This section will focus on starting short-acting hormonal contraceptives via telemedicine. Telemedicine visits for hormonal contraceptive initiation are most appropriate for adolescents who desire methods that do not require in-person procedures or administration, are reasonably not pregnant, and are not experiencing concerning symptoms (i.e., heavy bleeding or severe pelvic pain) [4]. Importantly, despite telemedicine's capacity to provide contraception initiation, patient preference should inform visit modality, with in-person visits still being offered.

Ruling Out Pregnancy

After a medically appropriate and desired contraceptive method is identified, the provider must be reasonably certain that the adolescent is not pregnant. Routine pregnancy testing is not necessary prior to initiating contraception; instead, providers can determine whether a patient is reasonably not pregnant through history (Table 7.3) [42]. If the provider cannot rule out a pregnancy, the benefits of initiating contraception generally outweigh the risks for all contraceptive methods, other than the IUD. In this situation, the healthcare provider should engage in shared decision-making with the adolescent to decide whether to start the contraceptive, offer

Table 7.3 Criteria to determine whether a patient is reasonably not pregnant [42]

The patient has no symptoms or signs of pregnancy *and* meets any one of the following: The patient…	
	is ≤7 days after the start of normal menses
	Has not had sexual intercourse since the start of last normal menses
	Has been correctly and consistently using a reliable method for contraception
	Is ≤7 days after spontaneous or induced abortion
	Is within 4 weeks postpartum
	Is fully or nearly fully breastfeeding, amenorrheic[a], and <6 months postpartum

These criteria are highly accurate for ruling out pregnancy (99–100% negative predictive value)
[a]Exclusively breastfeeding or breastfeeding for ≥85% of feeds

emergency contraception (if indicated), and recommend a pregnancy test (at home or in office) in 2–4 weeks [42].

Progesterone-Only Pills (POPs)

All progesterone-only pills (POPs) can be initiated at telemedicine visits. The US Selected Practice Recommendations (SPR) for Contraceptive Use does not recommend routine physical examinations or tests prior to initiating POPs [42]. A baseline BMI could be helpful to monitor for changes in weight over time [42]. Providers who wish to monitor for weight changes could use the documented weight from the last in-person visit or ask the patient for a self-reported weight. Initiation of POPs should not be delayed to obtain a baseline weight in clinic. If in line with the patient's preferences and anticipated use, the provider should prescribe a 1-year supply of POPs at the initial visit [4, 42].

Combined Hormonal Contraception (CHC)

All forms of combined hormonal contraception (CHC), including cOCPs, transdermal patches, and vaginal rings, can be initiated via telemedicine. The US SPR for Contraceptive Use recommends all patients have their blood pressure (BP) checked prior to initiating CHC given the elevated risks of stroke and myocardial infarction for those with hypertension who use an estrogen-containing method [42]. During a telemedicine visit, the provider can (1) use the most recent BP reading from an in-person visit within the previous 12 months; (2) request the patient check their BP at home or at a local pharmacy prior to method initiation; or (3) confirm the patient has no history of BP elevation, engage in a conversation about the risks of CHC use for people with hypertension, and schedule a non-urgent visit for a BP check [4, 42]. No other physical examination or testing is routinely recommended prior to starting CHC [42]. A baseline weight and BMI could be helpful to monitor for change over time [42]. Providers who wish to monitor for weight change could use the documented weight from the last in-person visit or ask the patient for a self-reported weight. Initiation of CHC should not be delayed to obtain a baseline weight in clinic. If in line with the patient's preferences and anticipated use, the provider should prescribe a 1-year supply of CHC at the initial visit [4, 42].

Depot Medroxyprogesterone Acetate (DMPA) Injection

DMPA can be initiated during a telemedicine visit if the patient desires DMPA via subcutaneous self-injection (DMPA-SC). The CDC and the World Health Organization support the use of DMPA-SC, in addition to DMPA-IM, given its potential to improve contraceptive access and increase patient autonomy [43]. It is important to note that the US FDA approved DMPA-SC in 2004 for administration by a healthcare professional; DMPA-SC administered via patient self-injection is an off-label use [44]. Therefore, the prescribing provider should use their clinical judgment to determine whether DMPA-SC is appropriate for their patient [44]. All clinics offering telemedicine sexual and reproductive health services should have procedures in place to help patients access and use DMPA-SC. If a patient prefers to receive DMPA administered by a clinician, an in-person visit will be required. A patient may wish to have a telemedicine visit to discuss DMPA-IM initiation, followed by a brief in-person visit for the injection [4]. Telemedicine DMPA consult visits should be optional, as required telemedicine visits prior to in-person DMPA-IM administration increase barriers to accessing desired contraceptive care.

The US SPR for Contraceptive Use does not recommend any routine physical exam or testing prior to DMPA initiation. A baseline weight and BMI could be helpful to monitor for changes over time [42]. Providers who wish to monitor weight could use the documented weight from the last in-person visit or ask the patient for a self-reported weight. Initiation of DMPA should not be delayed to obtain a baseline weight in clinic.

The provider reviews information from AG's most recent in-person clinic visit 5 months ago (BP 115/70 and BMI 28.5 kg/m². AG last had sex over a week ago and the first day of their last menstrual period was 5 days ago. The provider determines AG is reasonably not pregnant and it is appropriate to start the cOCP today. The provider reviews how to take the pills and potential side effects. The provider sends a 1-year supply of cOCPs to the pharmacy. AG asks when they need to see the provider again.

Contraception Surveillance

Telemedicine is considered an appropriate modality for contraceptive surveillance [2, 4, 8]. With the exception of annual BP monitoring for those using CHC, routine follow-up is not recommended for any contraceptive method. The evidence does not support routine weight surveillance for any method, routine arm examination for those using the implant, or routine pelvic examinations for those using the IUD [42]. Instead, all patients should be encouraged to return at any time to discuss side effects or a change in contraceptive method, if desired [42]. While the US SPR for Contraceptive Use asserts that adolescents may be a specific population that could benefit from closer contraceptive follow-up, [42] no formal guidelines for adolescent contraceptive surveillance exist. If performed, surveillance visits can be used to assess for side effects, method satisfaction, changes in health status or medications, and eligibility for the method. Telemedicine may be a useful modality for adolescent contraceptive surveillance.

An in-person contraceptive surveillance visit is most appropriate for a patient using any contraceptive method who is experiencing heavy bleeding, severe pelvic pain, or symptoms concerning for ectopic pregnancy (vaginal bleeding, pelvic pain, and/or positive pregnancy test) [4, 8]. For adolescents using the contraceptive implant, an in-person visit is indicated if the implant cannot be palpated. For adolescents using the IUD, an in-person visit is indicated for the evaluation of missing strings, suspected expulsion, or concern for pregnancy or positive pregnancy test given risk for ectopic pregnancy [4, 8]. If a patient reports any of these concerns during a telemedicine visit, the patient should be encouraged to seek care in-person as soon as possible.

While it is appropriate to offer a telemedicine visit to a patient who is interested in discussing side effects, requiring such a visit if the patient is requesting LARC removal is not appropriate. This practice would increase barriers to LARC removal and infringe on an individual's right to reproductive autonomy. It has been well established that patients seeking LARC removal experience coercion to keep their LARC device; [45–47] therefore, ensuring that adolescents have access to prompt LARC removal is paramount. Telemedicine LARC surveillance should only be used if in line with the adolescent's reproductive goals.

The provider tells AG that no routine follow-up visit is necessary and encourages AG to call to schedule a visit at any time to ask questions, discuss potential side effects, or change the method. The provider tells AG that follow-up visits could be virtual, as long as AG does not have heavy bleeding or severe pelvic pain. The provider reminds AG that annual BP monitoring is indicated while AG is taking the cOCPs and that this monitoring can be done at their annual routine health maintenance exam.

AG calls the clinic 10 months later to request a telemedicine follow-up visit with the provider. At that visit, AG reports that they were supposed to start a new pill pack 4 days ago but forgot until today. AG reports they took a pill today. AG reports unprotected sex yesterday. AG asks if they are protected against pregnancy.

Emergency Contraception (EC)

Emergency contraception (EC) options include oral pills and IUDs [42]. Oral EC can be provided via a virtual visit for patients who have had unprotected sex in the previous 5 days [4, 34]. For oral EC, providers can discuss provision of medication via prescription or over-the-counter based on laws in their practice area [48]. However, patients seeking an IUD for EC should be scheduled for an in-person visit for insertion within 5 days of unprotected sex. Of note, the use of the copper IUD or levonorgestrel 52 mg IUD is off label in the USA for EC.

Any of the available oral EC regimens can be recommended to adolescents via telemedicine. These options include ulipristal acetate 30 mg single dose, levonorgestrel 1.5 mg single dose, levonorgestrel as a split dose (0.75 mg initial dose followed by a second dose of 0.75 mg 12 h later), or cOCPs in two doses (one dose of 100 μg of ethinyl estradiol/0.50 mg of levonorgestrel followed by a second dose 12 h later) [42]. Of note, EC efficacy is impacted by BMI; levonorgestrel is most effective for people with BMI <26 kg/m^2, while ulipristal acetate is most effective for people with BMI <35 kg/m^2 [42]. Telemedicine may limit the ability to have the most recent weight or BMI measurement for a patient, which could in turn limit the provider's ability to give their best recommendation for EC choice. Providers can use the most recently documented BMI (if available) or ask for a patient's self-reported weight to help aid in decision-making. Patients should be counseled to take a pregnancy test if no withdrawal bleed occurs within 3 weeks following oral EC [42].

The provider tells AG that they are eligible for EC. After discussion, the provider prescribes AG levonorgestrel 1.5 mg as a single dose. The provider recommends continuing to take the cOCPs daily, to use a back-up contraceptive method for the next 7 days, and to take a pregnancy test within 3 weeks if no withdrawal bleed occurs.

Menstrual Management

Literature examining the use of telemedicine for menstrual management in adolescents is limited. One study described the use of telemedicine visits to address dysmenorrhea/endometriosis (n = 485), AUB (n = 225), amenorrhea (n = 20), and gender affirming care including hormonal management (n = 34) in pediatric and adolescent patients presenting to ambulatory care [28]. In this study, only one patient who was evaluated via telemedicine for a menstrual concern (listed above) presented for a subsequent visit in-person within the next 90 days. This finding suggests that the concerns were adequately addressed during the initial encounter for the majority of cases [28].

An in-person evaluation should be used for any patient experiencing heavy bleeding, severe pelvic pain, symptoms concerning for ectopic pregnancy, or symptoms of anemia [36]. If a patient with a complaint of AUB is seen via telemedicine, providers can observe the patient's general appearance (e.g., mentation, pallor, respirations) and may have the patient assist in the evaluation for hemodynamic stability. Patients can be guided to take their own vital signs (heart rate and blood pressure, depending on availability of equipment) and to perform certain physical examination steps (e.g., measuring capillary refill, assessing for conjunctival or oral pallor) [24]. Providers can ask about common symptoms of anemia (e.g., shortness of breath, dizziness, chest pain, headache, or lightheadedness). Providers can quantify bleeding by instructing the patient how to obtain a home sanitary pad weight or by visualizing the menstrual hygiene product (via photo or video) [24]. If additional evaluation is needed (e.g., laboratory testing or speculum exam), appropriate in-person follow-up should be arranged.

Hormonal agents are commonly used to manage these menstrual concerns. Providers can use the above guidelines and guidance for counseling and initiation of menstrual management options. A follow-up visit is likely indicated to ensure the intervention is successful in treating the identified concern.

Pregnancy

Telemedicine visits can be used to discuss concern for pregnancy and provide options counseling for a pregnant adolescent. While discussing the use of telemedicine for pregnancy care, including pre-natal, post-natal, and abortion care, is beyond the scope of this chapter, telemedicine has been utilized for these indications as well [2, 3, 34, 36, 37].

CW is a 17-year-old adolescent who calls the clinic to schedule an appointment to discuss concern for pregnancy. CW asks if the visit can be virtual because CW is not able to come to the clinic without a ride from their parent.

Evaluating for Pregnancy

Telemedicine visits can be used to help determine if someone is pregnant, provided that there is no concern for ectopic pregnancy (bleeding and/or pelvic pain) [33]. As previously mentioned, it is important to confirm that the adolescent is in a private space to safely have a confidential conversation about sexual history and potential pregnancy at the beginning of the visit. Providers can elicit a sexual history, menstrual history (including last menstrual period), and contraceptive history including the use of EC and assess for symptoms of pregnancy (such as nausea, fatigue, frequent urination, and breast tenderness) to determine likelihood of pregnancy. If pregnancy is possible based on history and the patient has not taken a pregnancy test, the provider can discuss options for pregnancy testing with the patient. It is important to recognize that it is not possible or preferable for all patients to acquire an over-the-counter pregnancy test and test outside the clinic. Many factors could influence this decision including cost of the test, concerns about buying a test in the store, lack of privacy, fear of parents finding the test, and wanting support interpreting results. Shared decision-making with the adolescent should be used to determine if urine pregnancy testing at home or in the clinic is the next best step.

If pregnancy is suspected, the provider should ask the adolescent about their feelings about a possible pregnancy and if they have considered what they would do if they were pregnant [49]. The provider could also assess support system, safety, and prior pregnancy history [49].

After triage with nursing staff to make sure CW is not experiencing bleeding or pelvic pain, CW is scheduled for a telemedicine visit to discuss concern for pregnancy. At this visit, the provider confirms CW is in a private space and feels comfortable discussing their sexual history and concern for pregnancy via telemedicine. CW reports consensual penile-vaginal sex 6 weeks ago without a barrier method. They are not currently using contraception. Last menstrual period was 8 weeks ago. Prior to this, CW's periods had always been regular (every 28 days). This week, CW started having nausea and breast tenderness. A couple of days after the sexual encounter, CW took a home urine pregnancy test and it was negative. CW asks if they should take another test. CW tells the provider they do not want to be pregnant, but they aren't sure what they would do if they were pregnant. CW reports their partner is supportive and knows about today's visit but is not sure how their parents will react. Despite concerns about discussing a potential pregnancy with their parents, CW reports feeling safe at home.

Pregnancy Test Interpretation

Urine pregnancy testing at home can be a useful tool during telemedicine visits. However, it is important to understand the limitations of at-home testing. Human error in performing the test can lead to false-negative or false-positive results [49]. A false-negative result can occur if the pregnancy test is taken too early (prior to the first day of the missed period), if the urine sample is dilute, or if the urine human chorionic gonadotropin (hCG) concentrations are extremely high (also known as the hook effect) [42, 49]. A false-positive result could occur for several weeks after an abortion because hCG levels may remain elevated [42]. Urine pregnancy tests done at home should be interpreted in the context of the clinical scenario. If clinical suspicion for pregnancy is high and the at-home urine pregnancy test is negative, the provider could recommend repeating the home test in several days or having the adolescent come into clinic for a urine or serum test [49].

The provider confirms that CW feels comfortable repeating the urine pregnancy test at home today. The visit is briefly paused for CW to perform the test. CW reports the urine pregnancy test is positive. CW asks what options are available.

Pregnancy Options Counseling

A discussion of pregnancy options can be offered via telemedicine [9]. Pregnancy options counseling may look different in telemedicine visits, as patients may be disclosing the results of an at-home pregnancy test during the visit, instead of the provider disclosing the results of a test done in clinic at an in-person visit. As with in-person pregnancy options counseling, the virtual discussion should be open-ended, non-judgmental, non-directive, and rooted in the fundamental principle that the adolescent has the answer as to which decision is best for them. The provider should discuss all options available to the adolescent including continuing the pregnancy and parenting, continuing the pregnancy and making a plan for adoption/kinship care, or having an abortion [49]. The provider should allow the adolescent sufficient time to make the decision that is right for them, recognizing the adolescent may decide during the first or subsequent encounters [49]. The provider should inquire whether the adolescent would like to include a support person(s) in the decision-making [49]. Once the adolescent has made their decision, the provider should facilitate appropriate referrals for prenatal or abortion care if needed, provide any additional resources needed (i.e., information about adoption or judicial bypass), and offer a follow-up visit to ensure the patient has successfully connected with appropriate clinical care and/or resources [49]. To date, few studies have assessed the use of telemedicine for pregnancy options counseling, with no studies assessing this practice specifically for adolescents. Therefore, further research is needed in this area, especially dedicated to the adolescent population.

The provider discusses all pregnancy options with CW. The provider answers all of CW's questions and facilitates next steps.

Conclusions

Sexual and reproductive health services are critical aspects of routine adolescent healthcare. In response to the COVID-19 pandemic, adolescent sexual and reproductive health telemedicine services were widely and rapidly implemented in an effort to maintain continuity and minimize disruptions to routine, essential clinical care. While advantages and disadvantages are inherent to these innovative methods of healthcare delivery, these modalities have generally been well received by both clinicians and patients.

In 2020, the North American Society for Pediatric and Adolescent Gynecology endorsed the use of telemedicine for adolescent reproductive healthcare [1]. This practice has also been recognized by the American Academy of Pediatrics and the American College of Obstetricians and Gynecologists as an appropriate alternative to traditional healthcare delivery methods (i.e., in-person office visits) with comparable health outcomes [2, 5].

Emerging research continues to explore the use of telemedicine for the provision of sexual and reproductive services for adolescents, including general counseling, contraception, STI testing and treatment, and various gynecological complaints. As the use of telemedicine increases, adequate planning and special attention to under-resourced populations are imperative in order to equitably expand access for those who face barriers to in-person care.

Despite its limitations, the use of telemedicine for sexual and reproductive health services may be an important tool to bridge the service gap for the delivery of healthcare, provided that principles for achieving health equity are used and carefully considered in its planning and execution. Clinicians who serve adolescent patients have an unprecedented opportunity to reexamine pre-pandemic practice patterns, increase patient-centered care, adopt evidence-based clinical practices, and decrease barriers to sexual and reproductive healthcare access. Evolving and adapting these practices to meet the needs of adolescents is key and has the potential for lasting impact for future generations. Continued evaluation of such innovations is thus necessary to understand how best to approach this essential care for adolescents.

References

1. Tyson N, Berlan E, Hewitt G. Provision of reproductive health for teens during a pandemic. J Pediatr Adolesc Gynecol. 2020;33:331.
2. ACOG Committe Opinion No. 798: implementing telehealth in practice. Obstet Gynecol. 2020;135:e73–e79.
3. Cohen MA, Powell AM, Coleman JS, Keller JM, Livingston A, Anderson JR. Special ambulatory gynecologic considerations in the era of coronavirus disease 2019 (COVID-19) and implications for future practice. Am J Obstet Gynecol. 2020;223:372–8.
4. Benson LS, Madden T, Tartelon J, Micks EA. Society of Family Planning interim clinical recommendations: contraceptive provision when healthcare access is restricted due to pandemic response–2021 update. Soc Family Plan. 2021:1–10.
5. Curfman A, McSwain SD, Chuo J, Yeager-McSwain B, Schinasi DA, Marcin J, et al. Pediatric telehealth in the COVID-19 pandemic era and beyond. Pediatrics. 2021;148:1–11.
6. Curfman AL, Hackell JM, Herendeen NE, Alexander JJ, Marcin JP, Moskowitz WB, et al. Telehealth: improving access to and quality of pediatric health care. Pediatrics. 2021;148:1–6.
7. Thompson TA, Sonalkar S, Butler JL, Grossman D. Telemedicine for family planning: a scoping review. Obstet Gynecol Clin N Am. 2020;47:287–316.
8. Wilkinson TA, Kottke MJ, Berlan ED. Providing contraception for young people during a pandemic is essential health care. JAMA Pediatr. 2020;174:823–4.
9. Telehealth FAQ for Preventive Care. In: Women's Preventive Services Initiative. 2018. https://www.womenspreventivehealth.org/faqs/. Accessed 3 Feb 2022.
10. Stifani BM, Avila K, Levi EE. Telemedicine for contraceptive counseling: an exploratory survey of US family planning providers following rapid adoption of services during the COVID-19 pandemic. Contraception. 2021;103:157–62.
11. Stifani BM, Smith A, Avila K, Boos EW, Ng J, Levi EE, et al. Telemedicine for contraceptive counseling: patient experiences during the early phase of the COVID-19 pandemic in New York City. Contraception. 2021;104:254–61.
12. Gilkey MB, Kong WY, Huang Q, Grabert BK, Thompson P, Brewer NT. Using telehealth to deliver primary care to adolescents during and after the COVID-19 pandemic: National Survey Study of US Primary Care Professionals. J Med Internet Res. 2021;23:e31240.
13. Toh N, Pawlovich J, Grzybowski S. Telehealth and patient-doctor relationships in rural and remote communities. Can Fam Physician. 2016;62:961–3.
14. Burke PJ, Coles MS, di Meglio G, Gibson EJ, Handschin SM, Lau M, et al. Sexual and reproductive health care: a position paper of the society for adolescent health and medicine references. J Adolesc Health. 2014;54:491–6.
15. Ross LJ, Solinger R. Reproductive justice: an introduction. Oakland: University of California Press; 2017.
16. Gilliam ML, Neustadt A, Gordon R. A call to incorporate a reproductive justice agenda into reproductive health clinical practice and policy. Contraception. 2009;79:243–6.
17. Ortega G, Rodriguez JA, Maurer LR, Witt EE, Perez N, Reich A, et al. Telemedicine, COVID-19, and disparities: policy implications. Health Policy Technol. 2020;9:368–71.
18. Hill BJ, Lock L, Anderson B. Racial and ethnic differences in family planning telehealth use during the onset of the COVID-19 response in Arkansas, Kansas, Missouri, and Oklahoma. Contraception. 2021;104:262–4.
19. Chen EM, Andoh JE, Nwanyanwu K. Socioeconomic and demographic disparities in the use of telemedicine for ophthalmic care during the COVID-19 pandemic. Ophthalmology. 2022;129:15–25.
20. Telemedicine Best Practices and Considerations. In: Partners in Contraceptive Choice and Knowledge (PICCK). https://picck.org/wp-content/uploads/2022/02/PICCK-Telemedicine-Best-Practices-and-Considerations.pdf. Accessed 7 Mar 2022.

21. Lewis R, Blake C, Shimonovich M, Coia N, Duffy J, Kerr Y, et al. Disrupted prevention: condom and contraception access and use among young adults during the initial months of the COVID-19 pandemic. An online survey. BMJ Sex Reprod Health. 2021;47:269–76.
22. FDA approves first injectable treatment for HIV pre-exposure prevention. In: U.S. Food & Drug Administration. 2021. https://www.fda.gov/news-events/press-announcements/fda-approves-first-injectable-treatment-hiv-pre-exposure-prevention. Accessed 18 May 2022.
23. Liddon N, Pampati S, Dunville R, Kilmer G, Steiner RJ. Annual STI testing among sexually active adolescents. Pediatrics. 2022;149:1–9.
24. Grimes CL, Balk EM, Dieter AA, et al. Guidance for gynecologists utilizing telemedicine during COVID-19 pandemic based on expert consensus and rapid literature reviews. Int J Gynaecol Obstet. 2020;150:288–98.
25. Sexually Transmitted Infections Treatment Guidelines, 2021. Centers for Disease Control and Prevention. 2021. https://www.cdc.gov/std/treatment-guidelines/chlamydia.htm. Accessed 15 Apr 2022.
26. Platt L, Elder H, Bassett I v, Molotnikov L, Klevens M, O'Connor E, et al. Chlamydia treatment practices and time to treatment in Massachusetts: directly observed therapy versus pharmacy prescriptions. J Prim Care Community Health. 2021;12:1–7.
27. Itriyeva K. Evaluation of vulvovaginitis in the adolescent patient. Curr Probl Pediatr Adolesc Health Care. 2020;50:1–9.
28. Shim JY, Kaur R, Laufer MR, Grimstad FW. The use of telemedicine in pediatric and adolescent gynecology. J Pediatr Adolesc Gynecol. 2022;35:133–7.
29. McKee M, Baquero M, Anderson M, Karasz A. Vaginal hygiene and douching: perspectives of Hispanic men. Cult Health Sex. 2009;11:159–71.
30. Brown JM, Poirot E, Hess KL, Brown S, Vertucci M, Hezareh M. Motivations for intravaginal product use among a cohort of women in Los Angeles. PLoS One. 2016;11:1–12.
31. Markham CM, Ph D, Tortolero SR, et al. Factors associated with frequent vaginal douching among alternative school youth. J Adolesc Health. 2007;41:509–12.
32. Francis JKR, Dapena L, Ma F, Catallozzi M, Rosenthal SL. Original study qualitative analysis of sexually experienced female adolescents: attitudes about vaginal health. J Pediatr Adolesc Gynecol. 2026;29:496–500.
33. American College of Obstetricians and Gynecologists. COVID-19 FAQs for obstetricians and gynecologists, gynecology. 2020. https://www.acog.org/clinical-information/physician-faqs/covid19-faqs-for-ob-gyns-gynecology. Accessed 3 Feb 2022.
34. Tolu LB, Feyissa TG, Jeldu WG. Guidelines and best practice recommendations on contraception and safe abortion care service provision amid covid-19 pandemic: scoping review. BMC Public Heath. 2021;21:1–10.
35. Holt K, Reed R, Crear-Perry J, Scott C, Wulf S, Dehlendorf C. Beyond same-day long-acting reversible contraceptive access: a person-centered framework for advancing high-quality, equitable contraceptive care. Am J Obstet Gynecol. 2020;222:S878.e1-S878.e6.
36. American College of Obstetricians and Gynecologists. COVID-19 FAQs for obstetrician–gynecologists, gynecology. 2020. https://www.acog.org/clinical-information/physician-faqs/covid19-faqs-for-ob-gyns-gynecology. Accessed 3 Feb 2022.
37. American College of Obstetricians and Gynecologists. COVID-19 FAQs for obstetricians-gynecologists, telehealth. 2020. https://www.acog.org/clinical-information/physician-faqs/covid-19-faqs-for-ob-gyns-telehealth. Accessed 3 Feb 2022.
38. American College of Obstetricians and Gynecologists. Patient-centered contraceptive counseling. Obstet Gynecol. 2022;139:350–3.
39. Shared Decision-making Approach to Contraceptive Counseling. Partners in Contraceptive Choice and Knowledge (PICCK). https://picck.org/wp-content/uploads/2022/01/PICCK-PICK-ONE-Infographic.pdf. Accessed 7 Mar 2022.
40. Centers for Disease Control and Prevention. US Medical Eligibility Criteria (US MEC) for Contraceptive Use, 2016. https://www.cdc.gov/reproductivehealth/contraception/mmwr/mec/summary.html. Accessed 16 May 2022.

41. Bryson A, Koyama A, Hassan A. Addressing long-acting reversible contraception access, bias, and coercion: supporting adolescent and young adult reproductive autonomy. Curr Opin Pediatr. 2021;33:345–53.
42. Curtis KM, Jatlaoui TC, Tepper NK, Zapata LB, Horton LG, Jamieson DJ, et al. U.S. selected practice recommendations for contraceptive use, 2016. MMWR Recomm Rep. 2016;65:1–66.
43. Curtis KM, Nguyen A, Reeves JA, Clark EA, Folger SG, Whiteman MK. Update to U.S. selected practice recommendations for contraceptive use: self-administration of subcutaneous depot medroxyprogesterone acetate. MMWR Recomm Rep. 2021;70:739–43.
44. National Family Planning & Reproductive Health Association. Self-administration of injectable contraception. 2020. https://www.nationalfamilyplanning.org/file/documents%2D%2D-service-delivery-tools/NFPRHA%2D%2D-Depo-SQ-Resource-guide%2D%2D-FINAL-FOR-DISTRIBUTION.pdf. Accessed 18 May 2022.
45. Amico JR, Bennett AH, Karasz A, Gold M. "I wish they could hold on a little longer": physicians' experiences with requests for early IUD removal. Contraception. 2017;96:106–10.
46. Amico JR, Bennett AH, Karasz A, Gold M. "She just told me to leave it": women's experiences discussing early elective IUD removal. Contraception. 2016;94:357–61.
47. Higgins JA, Kramer RD, Ryder KM. Provider bias in long-acting reversible contraception (LARC) promotion and removal: perceptions of young adult women. Am J Public Health. 2016;106:1932–7.
48. Guttmacher Institute. Emergency contraception. https://www.guttmacher.org/state-policy/explore/emergency-contraception#. Accessed 11 Jul 2022.
49. Hornberger LL, Breuner CC, Alderman EM, et al. Diagnosis of pregnancy and providing options counseling for the adolescent patient. Pediatrics. 2017;140:e20172273.

Chapter 8
Eating Disorder Care and Telemedicine

Jessica Van Huysse and Alana K. Otto

Introduction

Eating disorders are psychiatric disorders characterized by persistent disturbances of eating that lead to impaired health and/or psychosocial functioning [1]. These disorders are marked by distorted thoughts around eating, food, and/or body image; these thoughts lead to disordered behaviors, such as restricted and/or excessive intake of food, excessive exercise, and purging via self-induced vomiting or the misuse of laxatives, diuretics, or enemas; in turn, these behaviors lead to negative health and/or psychological consequences. The *Diagnostic and Statistical Manual of Mental Disorders, Fifth Edition* (DSM-5) names six specific eating disorders: anorexia nervosa, avoidant/restrictive food intake disorder (ARFID), binge eating disorder, bulimia nervosa, pica, and rumination disorder (Table 8.1); specific diagnostic criteria are outlined in the DSM-5. In addition, many patients with disordered eating do not meet the specific criteria for any named eating disorder and may be diagnosed with other specified feeding and eating disorders (OSFED) or an unspecified eating disorder.

Eating disorders are unique among psychiatric disorders in that they often lead to medical illness in addition to psychological symptoms. The medical consequences of eating disorders may be severe and in some cases life-threatening—indeed, eating disorders are associated with some of the highest mortality rates of all psychiatric disorders [2, 3], in part because of the risk for severe medical illness. Medical complications among individuals with eating disorders are primarily

J. Van Huysse
Department of Psychiatry, University of Michigan Medical School, Ann Arbor, MI, USA
e-mail: jvanhuy@med.umich.edu

A. K. Otto (✉)
Department of Pediatrics, University of Michigan Medical School, Ann Arbor, MI, USA
e-mail: alanako@med.umich.edu

Y. N. Evans et al. (eds.), *Telemedicine for Adolescent and Young Adult Health Care*, https://doi.org/10.1007/978-3-031-55760-6_8

Table 8.1 Specific eating disorder diagnoses and their clinical features

Diagnosis	Cardinal features
Anorexia nervosa	Intentional dietary restriction leading to weight loss, fear of weight gain, distorted perception of one's self as fat or overweight
Avoidant/restrictive food intake disorder	Avoidance of food related to sensory characteristics of food, lack of interest in eating, and/or fear of aversive consequences associated with eating (e.g., choking, abdominal pain)
Bulimia nervosa	Frequent episodes of binge eating and purging (e.g., intentional vomiting, misuse of laxatives, diuretics, or enemas)
Binge-eating disorder	Frequent episodes of binge eating without compensatory purging
Pica	Persistent and compulsive consumption of non-nutritive, non-food substances or objects
Rumination disorder	Persistent regurgitation of food

Table 8.2 Medical complications of malnutrition

Organ system	Effect(s) of malnutrition
Central nervous system	Brain atrophy, damage, and dysfunction related to specific nutrient deficiencies; mental fogginess; impaired memory and concentration; poor sleep; depressed mood
Autonomic nervous system	Orthostatic hypotension and/or tachycardia, postural dizziness, impaired temperature regulation
Endocrine	Hypothalamus-pituitary-adrenal axis dysfunction, hypogonadotropic hypogonadism, menstrual irregularities/amenorrhea, thyroid dysfunction, decreased bone mineral density
Cardiac	Myocardial atrophy, cardiac dysfunction, arrhythmias
Respiratory	Respiratory muscle wasting, exercise intolerance
Gastrointestinal	Liver dysfunction, gastroparesis, constipation, pancreatitis, superior mesenteric artery syndrome
Renal	Renal dysfunction, dehydration, electrolyte derangements
Hematologic	Bone marrow suppression, cytopenias
Integumentary	Telogen effluvium, poor wound healing, decubitus ulcers

related to fluid and electrolyte disturbances and/or to the sequelae of malnutrition. Clinically significant derangements of electrolytes, acid-base status, and/or fluid status may occur as a result of frequent vomiting or rumination, the misuse of laxatives, diuretics, or enemas, or among patients who consume excess water or other fluids to manipulate their weight or induce a sensation of satiety. Malnutrition affects all body systems and may lead to numerous manifestations of end-organ dysfunction (see Table 8.2). Patients with significant fluid and/or electrolyte abnormalities and/or those with signs and symptoms of severe malnutrition are at risk for medical decompensation and may require inpatient medical admission for stabilization. The Society for Adolescent Health and Medicine has published criteria for inpatient medical admission for adolescents with eating disorders, including physiologic instability (e.g., heart rate < 50 beats per minute while awake, blood pressure < 90/40 mm Hg, or temperature < 35.6 °C), electrolyte derangements, acute medical complications of malnutrition (e.g., syncope), uncontrolled purging, BMI

<75% of the median for age and sex, acute food refusal of ≥24 h, and failure of outpatient treatment [4]. In addition to severe medical illness, individuals with eating disorders are at increased risk for suicidal ideation, suicide attempts, and death by suicide, relative to the general population [2, 5–8].

Traditionally, eating disorders—particularly anorexia nervosa and bulimia nervosa—have been described as primarily affecting young women, with those of white race and high socioeconomic status overrepresented relative to the general population; however, eating disorders affect people of all genders, races/ethnicities, and socioeconomic circumstances [9–11]. Although ARFID, pica, and rumination disorder can occur at any age, childhood onset is most common. Conversely, anorexia nervosa, bulimia nervosa, and binge-eating disorder are uncommon in prepubertal children and most commonly begin in adolescence or young adulthood [1]. Clinicians should be aware of red flags for disordered eating thoughts and behaviors in adolescents (Table 8.3) and consider an eating disorder in the differential diagnosis of adolescent patients with weight loss, electrolyte derangements, and/or changes in eating patterns regardless of their gender, race/ethnicity, or socioeconomic status.

The treatment of eating disorders involves both prompt medical care to address any medical complications and psychotherapy to address disordered thoughts and behaviors. Treatment typically involves an interdisciplinary team of medical providers, therapists, dietitians, and/or psychiatrists. Family-based treatment (FBT) and enhanced cognitive behavioral therapy (CBT-E) are two therapeutic approaches that have an evidence base for use in children and adolescents and are the most frequently studied in telehealth formats. Below we briefly review the core components of these treatments as they were originally designed for in-person care.

Family-based treatment is a first-line intervention for anorexia nervosa, with some evidence for use with bulimia nervosa, ARFID, and OSFED [12]. FBT is an outpatient treatment that is typically delivered across 20 psychotherapy sessions over 6–12 months. The treatment incorporates parents or other caregivers as key in helping their child recover from the eating disorder and is divided into three phases. During the first phase, parents are given responsibility for decisions about what and

Table 8.3 Red flags for disordered eating behaviors in adolescents

Weight loss, weight gain, or weight fluctuations; failure to gain weight as expected (decreasing weight and/or BMI percentiles for age)

Abrupt and/or significant changes in eating patterns
  Avoiding foods one used to enjoy
  Avoiding entire food groups
  Skipping meals or snacks
  Eating different foods than the rest of the family
  Eating alone; refusing to eat in front of family/others

Distress or anxiety if expectations or routines around food change
Excessive or compulsive exercise; distress if asked or required to skip exercise
Food going missing; consuming large amounts of food at night or in secrecy
Repeatedly using the restroom immediately after meals; spending an unusual amount of time in the restroom

how much their child needs to eat, and they are asked to supervise all meals and snacks. For children who need to restore weight, parents are asked to serve the amount of food they know their malnourished child needs. Regardless of the need for weight restoration, parents are encouraged to reincorporate all foods the child ate prior to the eating disorder. For instance, if their child previously loved macaroni and cheese but cut it out due to fear of the calorie and fat content, parents would be encouraged to reintegrate this food by routinely preparing it, serving it, and sitting with their child to supervise the meal. Parents are also tasked with supporting their child by interrupting other eating disorder behaviors, such as binge eating, purging, laxative or diuretic misuse, excessive exercise, and caloric restriction. This is usually accomplished via increased supervision and communication. Phase two of FBT involves the gradual reintroduction of decisions about eating to the child, while parents still protect them from reverting to disordered behaviors. Alongside this there is also a gradual decrease in parental supervision of meals as the child shows the ability to eat adequately without it. During phase three, families focus on returning to the normative issues and concerns that typically arise during this time. FBT is considered a first-line treatment approach and results in significant improvements in symptoms for most children and adolescents with eating disorders. For instance, a review of the randomized controlled trials of FBT for anorexia nervosa indicated an average of about 75% of adolescents with anorexia nervosa demonstrate improvements in weight and eating disorder symptoms [13]. However, rates of full recovery are less than optimal (e.g., <40%; [13]).

Enhanced cognitive behavioral therapy (CBT-E) is an alternate treatment that is transdiagnostic, meaning it is modifiable for use with all eating disorder diagnoses [14]. CBT-E differs from FBT in that it aims to engage the patient in treatment and help them decide to make changes to their behaviors, rather than tasking their parents with managing the illness [14]. CBT-E is primarily completed in an outpatient setting, and the adolescent version is divided into three stages. The first stage is focused on psychoeducation, engaging the patient in treatment, and the patient beginning to make behavioral changes (e.g., establishing a pattern of regular eating). The second stage continues the interventions from the first stage while also addressing cognitive symptoms such as body image and dietary restraint. The third stage includes sessions on maintaining change and relapse prevention [14]. Although most studies of CBT-E to date have focused on adults, there is a growing evidence base for use in adolescents with anorexia nervosa and other eating disorders, with data indicating up to 65% of adolescents with anorexia nervosa demonstrate weight normalization after treatment and 68% of adolescents with non-underweight eating disorders demonstrate minimal eating disorder symptoms at the end of treatment [14].

Historically, medical and psychological care for eating disorders has taken place in the in-person setting. While some data on the use of digital psychotherapy interventions (including telehealth, application or "app" based, and virtual reality services) existed prior to the year 2020, the COVID-19 pandemic and its associated public health precautions sparked a significant and rapid shift to telemedicine eating disorder services across the globe [15–20]. Beyond the circumstances of the pandemic, transitioning treatments to telehealth provides a promising opportunity to improve access to evidence-based care by reducing or eliminating geographical constraints [21, 22]. Emerging evidence indicates telemedicine may be successfully utilized for eating disorder care, particularly psychotherapy services; however, there remains a paucity of data on the use of telemedicine to treat individuals with eating disorders.

Medical Care for Eating Disorders Via Telemedicine

Case 1

Sarah is a 16-year-old cisgender woman who presents to her primary care pediatrician for an urgent telemedicine visit with a chief complaint of weight loss. She is accompanied to the visit by her mother. Throughout the visit, Sarah is resistant to appearing on camera and defers most of the history to her mother.

Sarah's mother reports she noticed a change in Sarah's eating and exercise habits approximately 6 months ago; initially, the mother did not think much of the changes other than to be pleased with her daughter's efforts to be "healthier." One week ago, during a family vacation, Sarah's mother became concerned Sarah had lost a significant amount of weight when she saw her in a bathing suit for the first time in approximately 1 year; mother describes Sarah as looking "like skin and bones." Over the last week, Sarah's mother has tried to encourage her to eat more, but Sarah has eaten very little, telling her mother she is not hungry. Sarah's mother has also noticed Sarah spending an usual amount of time in the bathroom over the last week.

Sarah seems reluctant to answer questions about eating or to discuss her weight or eating habits. She again reports she has not been eating much because she is "not hungry." She does not answer most direct questions about how she has been feeling physically, but her mother endorses recent signs of fatigue, presyncope, irritability, and cold intolerance. Mother also thinks Sarah has been constipated and has not had a menstrual period in the last few months. Neither Sarah nor her mother knows how much she weighs, as they do not have a scale at home.

The pediatrician recommends Sarah present to the office for an in-person appointment to check a weight and vital signs as soon as possible. The next day, she is seen in the office, where she is noted to have lost 17 kg (37 pounds) since her most recent well-child examination 8 months prior and to have significant bradycardia and hypotension with a heart rate of 42 beats per minute and blood pressure 82/42 mmHg. She appears cachectic and frail with a body mass index of 13 kg/m^2 (less than the first percentile for age). During private interview with the pediatrician, she reluctantly endorses intentional restriction, fear of weight gain, and a distorted perception of her body as fat; she also endorses inducing vomiting up to *four times per day with a goal of losing weight. She is diagnosed with anorexia nervosa and admitted to the inpatient pediatrics service at a local hospital for medical stabilization given her bradycardia, hypotension, and uncontrolled purging.*

Traditionally, medical care for individuals with eating disorders has taken place almost exclusively in the in-person setting; there is little to no data on medical care delivered via telemedicine for this population published prior to the year 2020. Early in the COVID-19 pandemic, some institutions described rapid implementation of telemedicine services, including medical care, for eating disorder patients as public health precautions related to the pandemic resulted in restricted or limited availability of in-person medical care [23, 24]. These reports suggest medical care via telemedicine may be feasible for adolescents with eating disorders; however, there remains a paucity of data on outcomes, and evidence-based recommendations for implementing virtual medical care for adolescents with eating disorders are lacking.

The medical care of adolescents with eating disorders typically involves assessment and ongoing monitoring of weight, vital signs (e.g., temperature, heart rate, blood pressure), and physical examination findings; some patients may also need to have laboratory studies (e.g., electrolytes) monitored. For many patients, it may be feasible to measure weights at home; practical and psychological considerations related to monitoring weights at home are discussed in further detail below. In some cases, it may be more appropriate to have patients present for an in-person visit to check weight—for example, if there is concern for weight manipulation and/or medical instability. Although some authors have described strategies for measuring vital signs at home [24], home monitoring of vital signs has been discouraged by others, as patients and their caregivers often have not been trained to measure and/or interpret vital signs, and values obtained at home may not be accurate [25]. Vital signs should therefore be measured by an appropriately trained healthcare professional whenever possible, and providers may consider the potential limitations when recommending home vital sign monitoring and/or when using vital sign measurements obtained at home to guide clinical decision-making. In general, laboratory studies must be collected in a clinical setting. Thus, in most cases, patients with eating disorders will need to be seen in-person at least periodically for medical monitoring, and in-person evaluation remains the standard of care for medical visits for adolescents with eating disorders. Collaboration and creativity may be utilized, particularly for patients who live in remote areas with limited access to subspecialty medical care for eating disorders; for example, an adolescent with anorexia nervosa who lives in a rural area may see a medical provider with expertise in eating disorders located several hundred miles away exclusively via telemedicine and see their local primary care provider for weight checks, vital signs, and laboratory studies, the results of which may be shared electronically with the eating disorder specialist.

Privacy and confidentiality are paramount to adolescent healthcare. Although eating disorder care for adolescents rarely happens entirely confidentially, some aspects of the medical care of adolescents with eating disorders may involve private conversations between the clinician and the patient or between the clinician and the patient's caregiver(s). In particular, information that may be distressing to the patient, such as weights and/or recommendations regarding calories, often needs to be transmitted between a patient's caregiver(s) and their medical provider; depending on the patient's course of illness and recovery status, such information may not be shared with the patient directly. Medical providers caring for adolescents with eating disorders via telemedicine should be familiar with strategies for communicating with patients and/or caregivers privately; these strategies are described in detail elsewhere (see Chap. 2 on confidentiality).

Medical providers caring for adolescents with eating disorders via telemedicine must also be prepared to address urgent medical and/or psychiatric concerns that arise during telemedicine visits. Patients who report concerning physical or psychiatric symptoms (e.g., syncope or presyncope, chest pain, uncontrolled vomiting, suicidality) during telemedicine visits should be seen urgently for in-person evaluation. Patients may need to be directed to their primary care provider or local emergency room if located far from the provider they are seeing virtually, or if the telemedicine provider does not have the capacity to see them in an appropriate time frame. Additionally, telemedicine providers should be familiar with indications for medical admission, such those outlined by Golden et al. [4], and standards of care for emergent medical evaluation and/or inpatient medical admission should be followed regardless of whether a patient is seen via telemedicine or in person [25].

Psychotherapy for Eating Disorders Via Telemedicine

Case 2: Part 1

Jack is a 15-year-old white, cisgender male whose parents bring him to his pediatrician after walking in on him during an episode of self-induced vomiting at home. During the pediatrician visit, Jack discloses weekly episodes of binge eating and purging via self-induced vomiting, episodes of fasting, and compulsive exercise patterns (e.g., waking up at 5 am to secretly engage in exercises in his bedroom for 60 minutes each day before school). Jack reports these symptoms started about 6 months ago and that he has wanted some help but felt embarrassed about what was happening. He has continued to make expected weight gains for development, and his BMI is at the 60th BMI percentile for age, which is consistent with his historical growth trajectory. Jack reports that he is preoccupied with negative thoughts about his body shape and weight and feels driven to check his body by looking in the mirror; he has also been weighing himself multiple times daily. He reports feeling down and depressed every time he sees the number on the scale, noting it makes him feel guilty and "like a failure." Jack does not present with any vital sign or laboratory abnormalities that would suggest a need for an intensive level of care or hospitalization, and thus outpatient psychotherapy and ongoing medical monitoring are recommended.

The pediatrician specifically recommends Jack to seek outpatient family-based treatment (FBT). However, Jack lives in a rural area of the state, and there are no therapists near his home that have any experience with eating disorders. Fortunately, the pediatrician is aware of an in-state treatment team that offers virtual evidence-based eating disorder treatment. Jack and his family schedule a virtual intake the following week. In addition to arranging virtual FBT, regular medical visits are scheduled so that weight, vital signs, and laboratory tests can be monitored. Release of information forms are signed so the FBT team and the pediatrician can communicate directly regarding Jack's progress.

Outpatient Eating Disorder Psychotherapy Via Telemedicine

Treatment Effectiveness

Eating disorder treatment via telemedicine was relatively rare prior to the COVID-19 pandemic, with only a few empirical studies—primarily small case series or case studies—discussing the topic. For instance, three small studies that included 2–12 participants each examined cognitive behavioral therapy (CBT) for adults who were primarily diagnosed with bulimia nervosa, binge eating disorder, or OSFED; these studies demonstrated the treatment approach was feasible via telehealth and suggested some promising clinical improvements, such as reduced eating disorder symptoms [26–30]. A telemedicine relapse prevention study of 16 adults with anorexia nervosa who were stepping down from a higher level of care suggested the intervention was safe, feasible, and acceptable to the patients and may have contributed to maintenance of change or symptom improvement [31]. A larger ($n = 128$) randomized trial comparing CBT for bulimia nervosa in adults via face-to-face versus virtual modalities found generally similar improvements in eating disorder and depression symptoms across modalities, though there were some marginal findings in favor of face-to-face treatment, such as a slightly larger reduction in eating disorder cognitions and depression symptoms in the face-to-face treatment group [32].

The literature specific to adolescents and teletherapy for eating disorders prior to the COVID-19 pandemic was even more sparse than the literature on adults, with just two empirical articles published on the topic: one case study of the use of virtual family therapy in an adolescent with anorexia nervosa [33] and a study aimed to develop and examine the feasibility of FBT for youth with anorexia nervosa in a sample of ten adolescents [34, 35]. Findings supported the feasibility of virtual FBT, with good retention in treatment and improvements in BMI and self-reported eating disorder symptoms [34].

As with many other mental health diagnoses, virtual treatment for youth with eating disorders rapidly increased in 2020, when clinics around the world rapidly transitioned to telehealth care models due to COVID-19 (see Chap. 10 on mental health). The transition to telehealth also led to more research on the effectiveness of virtual psychotherapy for youth with eating disorders. Though these studies were not designed to be randomized trials of virtual versus face-to-face treatment, the accumulating observational studies of outcomes associated with telehealth in the context of COVID-19 are promising. For instance, one study examined outcomes in 25 individuals between the ages of 16 and 47 who initiated treatment prior to COVID-19 and shifted to virtual care due to the pandemic. Participants were diagnosed with anorexia nervosa, bulimia nervosa, or another specified/unspecified eating disorder and received either FBT (if under age 18) or CBT-E (if over age 18). Patients treated via telehealth achieved similar outcomes compared to a cohort that received in-person treatment prior to the pandemic, and examination of within-person treatment progress suggested similar treatment effectiveness following the transition to telehealth at the onset of the pandemic [36]. A similar study in adults examined patients receiving outpatient treatment for eating disorders via telehealth due to COVID-19 compared to a pre-pandemic cohort that received traditional face-to-face care. Patients primarily had diagnoses of anorexia nervosa, bulimia nervosa, or OSFED, with a smaller proportion of patients having diagnoses of ARFID, and their outpatient treatment involved weekly group therapy, bimonthly individual therapy, and additional nutrition and pharmacological consultations based on patient need. Results suggested similar improvements in eating disorder symptoms and BMI, as well as similar treatment satisfaction, between the in-person and virtual treatment cohorts [37]. Other small-case studies of FBT delivered via telehealth have also suggested positive outcomes [38]. The only study to date focused on virtual interventions for ARFID included 15 individuals with severe ARFID (ages 2–7.5 years) who participated in an intensive in-person day treatment feeding program and then received outpatient follow-up for ARFID that was either in-person or virtual. Findings suggested equivalent outcomes for face-to-face compared to virtual treatment [39]. Together, findings since the onset of COVID-19 generally support the earlier pre-pandemic literature, suggesting that eating disorder psychotherapy delivered via telehealth is likely effective in reducing eating disorder and related symptoms in youth. However, the literature on delivery of evidence-based treatments via telehealth remains sparse, and larger trials are needed to recommend telehealth interventions more conclusively [25]. Some such studies are currently underway, such as a multi-site implementation study of virtual FBT, which will aim to assess treatment fidelity to in-person FBT, participant experiences with virtual FBT, and treatment outcomes [40].

Patient and Provider Experience of Telehealth

In addition to the likely clinical effectiveness of telehealth interventions, there is also evidence to suggest patients and providers broadly report satisfaction with provision of eating disorder care via telehealth. For instance, patients who participated in the randomized trial of CBT for bulimia nervosa for adults rated therapeutic alliance and technique similarly across in-person versus virtual treatment modalities, suggesting the telehealth format did not reduce the patient's perception of the therapeutic alliance [41]. In a small survey ($n = 25$) of adolescent and adult patients treated virtually during COVID-19, telehealth was rated "as good" or "better than" in-person care in most cases (76% of participants), and likewise, the therapeutic relationship during virtual care was rated "as good as usual" by a majority of participants (88%; [36]). In another study, youth and their parents receiving eating disorder treatment virtually in the context of COVID-19 were asked to rate their experience of virtual therapy in questions assessing their overall experience, feeling understood, whether the therapy addressed important issues, the impact of technology, and if they benefitted from online treatment, and overall impressions from both the youth and their parents were positive [42]. However, there have also been reports of patient concerns with virtual therapy, including a sense that there is "something lost" via virtual care in terms of building rapport and feeling connected to the therapist as well as the ability to pick up on body language or other nuances in expression [42]. In a qualitative study of adults receiving online therapy for eating disorders, many participants reported they formed strong therapeutic relationships with their therapists and appreciated the ease of attending sessions virtually, but there were also concerns of feeling less connected to the therapist and difficulty sharing openly due to concerns about confidentiality when other family members were home [43]. A study that asked patients to rank-order preferences for in-person versus telephone versus video appointments largely rated in-person as their top preference, though service satisfaction was not any lower during the period of COVID-19 (when most care provision was virtual) compared to prior to the pandemic [18]. In one study of adolescents and adults with eating disorders completed early in the COVID-19 pandemic, most patients indicated that they would prefer not to continue online (68%) and would not recommend it (54%); [16]. Overall, it appears though most patients can adapt to telehealth and that symptom improvements are observed in this context, there remain patients who prefer in-person care and may experience a negative effect on the therapeutic relationship with their therapist with virtual care [44, 45]. In the studies that were conducted in the midst of the most acute period of the COVID-19 pandemic, some of the negative impressions of virtual care may have been impacted by the rapid transition to this modality with a lack of preparation and training for the healthcare system and therapist, though this has not been directly examined. Providers also sometimes report concerns with the provision of virtual therapies, such as difficulty building rapport with patients with EDs virtually, a sense that monitoring patient status is more challenging remotely, concerns that the virtual treatment is ineffective, and specific challenges related to eating disorder care, such as supervising meals [25, 42, 46], though others have suggested that many of these concerns can be managed with planning and making small adjustments [38, 47].

Implementation of Eating Disorder Psychotherapy Via Telehealth

Overall, findings support the use of telemedicine to provide therapy to youth with eating disorders as a reasonable alternative to in-person care, particularly in circumstances when traditional in-person care is inaccessible [44]. Many elements of the psychotherapies typically used to treat eating disorders transition well into the telehealth format. For instance, a primary aim of FBT is for the therapist to assist parents in managing the eating disorder behaviors, and since parents remain with their child in the context of virtual FBT, the parental day-to-day parental management of the illness may be quite similar in the virtual treatment context. Similarly, clinicians have noted that many aspects of CBT-E, such as the cognitive work, can be transitioned quite well to virtual care [48]. However, there are some specific challenges relevant to virtual eating disorder care, which are discussed below.

Weight Monitoring Evidence-based psychotherapies for eating disorders typically involve assessment of weight at each psychotherapy session, which is done at the therapist's office during traditional in-person care. In the context of virtual care, different arrangements need to be made, which can include weight checks using a home scale or weight checks at a local physician office [22, 47]. Home weights require attention and planning surrounding a few concerns that may emerge in the context of eating disorder treatment. Having access to a scale at home can present some challenges, since individuals with eating disorders often engage in unhelpful weight checking behaviors (e.g., checking weight daily or multiple times daily). In the context of in-person psychotherapy, it is not uncommon for clinicians to recommend that patients remove scales from their homes and only see their weight at each weekly therapy appointment. Given the need to have home scale access during virtual treatment, the therapist needs to discuss with the patient/family how to obtain a weekly weight at home without encouraging excessive weight checking. If the patient is unable to resist urges to check weight between sessions, solutions can be explored, such as a family member hiding the scale between appointments. In some situations, patients with eating disorders may also have urges to report an inaccurate weight to the clinician, for example, wanting to convey that they are a higher weight than they are to avoid hospitalization. This can be managed by asking a family member to view the weight with the patient, particularly in the context of FBT, when the parents likely will be managing the weight checks with their child [47]; alternatively, additional weight and vitals checks may be conducted in person locally with the patient's primary care provider and reported directly to the virtual psychotherapist [47]. It has also been recommended that the patient/family obtain the weight just before or during the session, as this replicates the typical in-person procedure, where weight is usually obtained at the start of the session, allowing the therapist to respond in the moment to patient reactions to the weight [48]. Both FBT and CBT-E involve reviewing weight charts, which plot the patient's weight trajectory, with the patient/family; this can be accomplished virtually by holding a paper graph up to the screen, via screen share features, or otherwise sent to the family electronically [40, 47, 48]. Some patients who are weighed both at the physician's office and on a home scale at different times may be sensitive to small weight changes that may be attributable to differences in scale readings; the therapist can review with the patient that scales differ [48], and this may even provide context to reinforce that minor changes in weight are unhelpful to focus on.

In-Session Eating Eating disorder psychotherapy sometimes involves the patient/ family eating during the session. In FBT, the second session of the treatment is a family meal, where the family is asked to bring a meal that is chosen by the caregivers and includes foods they know their child needs (i.e., is not chosen based upon eating disorder preferences). The therapist then aims to help the parents identify strategies to get their child to eat more than they were initially willing to eat. In individual treatment, food-related exposures are sometimes completed during the session. In the context of virtual therapy, it has been noted that it may be especially difficult for the therapist to make the same observations about the content of the meal and eating disorder behaviors (e.g., hiding foods) that can be observed in person [47]. Given these challenges, it has been suggested that the therapist be especially attentive to working with the patient/family to position the camera in a way that enhances the view of the meal and patient eating and that the therapist may need to ask more explicit questions about the food served [47]. Some advantages of virtual in-session eating have also been noted, such as the therapist being able to observe the patient/family eating in their home environment and explicitly discuss changes from before/during the eating disorder, easy access to additional food (e.g., if the patient discards part of the meal, it can be replaced), and helping parents build confidence to renourish in the home environment (versus attributing success to the clinic) and may even easily invite discussion of the impact of pets on eating, for example, if there are eating disorder urges to secretly feed some of the meal to the family dog [47].

Privacy Ensuring patient privacy is relevant for telehealth in general, such as using an appropriate technology platform that allows secure virtual connections and ensuring that the patient has a private location to talk. Taking care with these issues can be important in helping patients and families feel comfortable to share, as feeling a lack of privacy in the home (e.g., fear that family members or roommates will overhear discussions) is often described as a reason for not preferring telehealth in qualitative studies [42]. In the context of treatment for eating disorders, especially when both a patient and caregivers are involved in treatment, privacy can be especially important to address. For instance, in FBT, the patient typically has a private check-in with therapist at the start of the session. In another form of FBT, called separated FBT, the parents participate without the patient present [12]. The therapist will need to discuss with the family how they can minimize chances that others will overhear. In separated FBT, patients may be curious to know the content of parent sessions, and families should be aware that their child may try to listen intentionally. The therapist can help to ensure conversations are private using strategies recommended to protect privacy in telehealth more generally, such as by asking directly whether the patient/family is in a private space or utilizing other strategies such as headphones or asking the patient/family to take their device to a more private location [47].

In-Session Behaviors When working with youth with eating disorders, there can be behavioral escalations that occur during the session, such as a patient becoming emotionally dysregulated, expressing safety concerns, or abruptly leaving the session by walking away or disconnecting the video [47]. It is important that therapists develop a plan to manage these issues, including having contact information for a parent/caregiver to reach them if these behaviors occur when parents are not part of the session. When parents are involved in the session and these behaviors occur, the therapist can work with the parents to ensure safety concerns are addressed and support parent management of behaviors [47]. It has also been noted that patients with eating disorders may be especially sensitive to viewing their own image during the video call due to body image concerns. This can be managed by allowing the patient to hide their image on the screen using application settings [49] or to participate by voice initially, and more on-screen time can be encouraged using exposure-based strategies [47].

Involving Multiple Family Members One benefit of telehealth is that it may increase the ease with which multiple family members can attend appointments [50, 51]. Indeed, though it is likely best for the family to be in the same space during FBT, attendance of all family members can be facilitated by allowing individuals to log-in to the visit from multiple locations (e.g., one parent joining from work). This can also more easily allow individuals from multiple households to participate, such as divorced parents and each of their new partners [52]. During sessions involving multiple participants, it is important for the therapist to facilitate a seating arrangement most conducive to family members interacting with one another as well as the therapist. Without this guidance, families may seat themselves such that they are all looking at the screen rather than one another, which may hamper crosstalk among the family [47].

Case 2: Part 2

During Jack's initial therapy appointment, the therapist provides an overview of FBT and asks the family to share their observations on the impact of the eating disorder on Jack and the family. The central role Jack's parents will play in his recovery is discussed, and the importance of consistent attendance of family members is highlighted. The therapist tasks Jack's parents with serving food regularly (three meals and two snacks daily) and asks them to choose, portion, and supervise all meals and snacks. The therapist also asks parents to help Jack to reduce binge eating, purging, fasting, and excessive exercise behaviors with increased supervision and redirection of these behaviors. The therapist asks Jack to keep a log of any purging or binge eating episodes that do occur. Jack's parents are asked to monitor his weight at home via *weekly weight checks with the home scale on the day of therapy appointments. Jack's parents are concerned about bringing the scale back to the home, as the pediatrician suggested they remove it in response to Jack's weight-checking behaviors. The therapist reinforced that this is a common and sensible recommendation; however, in the context of virtual care, it will be important to have weekly weight updates during therapy sessions. Ultimately, the parents and therapist decide that they can meet both goals by arranging to keep the scale at his mother's office and bring it home only on the days they check weight.*

The therapist replicates the structure of in-person FBT within the telehealth format as much as feasible, including completing a private check-in with Jack for the first few minutes of each session. The therapist and the family jointly identify the best location in their home to complete sessions, where each family member can sit such that they see the therapist on the screen and one another; they settle on the family sitting on the couch with the laptop positioned on the coffee table. Since both parents are adjusting their work schedules to support Jack, one parent often goes to the office while the other stays at home with Jack. With the virtual care model, the working parent occasionally participates in treatment sessions from the office during their lunch hour when they are unable to return home for the appointment.

With the guidance of the therapist, the family effectively progresses through the three phases of FBT over the course of about 13 months. The therapist finds that most elements of manualized FBT are possible to implement via *video. There are some challenges with the video format that are addressed, such as Jack feeling reluctant to share openly during one-on-one time due to a concern that other family members may overhear the discussion, which is remedied by identifying a specific location in the home where Jack feels less likely to be overheard, combined with the use of headphones. During two sessions in the beginning of treatment, Jack becomes overwhelmed by the discussion about increasing bathroom supervision to prevent additional purging episodes, and he abruptly leaves the session. The therapist and parents discuss how best to manage the departures from the session while also making sure Jack is safe. They settle on one parent checking on Jack while the other parent continues the session, and Jack is able to regulate and return within a few minutes on both occasions.*

The first phase of treatment takes about 4 months, during which parents are given the responsibility of making decisions about what Jack eats and interrupting all of Jack's eating disorder symptoms. Jack notices that his urges to binge eat start to decrease rather rapidly as he starts to eat three meals and two snacks during the day, quite different from his previous pattern of trying to restrict during the day. His parents also work on challenging his food rules, such as serving foods that Jack previously liked that were reduced or cut out in the context of the eating disorder, either due to fears of bingeing on them, or fears that they are too "unhealthy." Jack starts to see some of the benefits of challenging his eating disorder behaviors directly, begins to become more engaged in the treatment process, and even independently challenges himself on some occasions. As Jack makes progress, the family describes a gradual decrease in the intensity of eating disorder behaviors and cognitions, though body image concerns remain prominent for many months. After about 4 months, Jack is no longer engaging in binge eating or purging episodes and reports minimal urges, meals are progressing smoothly, and Jack's parents report confidence in managing his eating disorder urges and behaviors. The family and FBT therapist move forward through phases two and three of FBT over the next 9 months, gradually supporting Jack with more independence regarding food selection while continuing to utilize parental supervision and support to prevent eating disorder behaviors. By the end of treatment, Jack is choosing his meals and snacks independently, continuing his abstinence from binge eating and purging episodes, is no longer engaging in excessive exercise (though he has begun to participate on his school soccer team), and has incorporated all foods that he ate prior to the eating disorder. He describes transient body image concerns, but they do not disrupt his functioning. During the last psychotherapy session, the family expresses appreciation for their FBT therapist and remarks that they have felt connected and supported despite interacting exclusively via telehealth.

Use of Telehealth for Eating Disorder Treatment in Higher Levels of Care

Though traditional outpatient psychotherapy is perhaps most directly adaptable to telehealth, some people with eating disorders require higher levels of care to interrupt symptoms. This can include intensive outpatient programs (IOP), which typically involve attending treatment at least 3 h/day, 3 days/week, or partial hospitalization programs (PHP; typically 5–7 days a week for 6+ h/day). Both intensive outpatient and partial hospitalization programs typically integrate group therapy, individual and/or family therapy, and nutritional interventions and meal support, though the specific components of individual programs vary considerably. For individuals needing even more intensive support, residential programs, which often last 1–3 months and provide 24/7 monitoring in addition to the types of interventions described above, are available. Individuals requiring the highest level of stabilization may require medical or psychiatric hospitalization. Further details about the clinical indications for each level of care are available elsewhere [53], as we focus specifically on telehealth adaptations in these levels of care.

Intensive Outpatient and Partial Hospitalization Programs

Few studies have examined the implementation of telehealth in partial hospitalization and intensive outpatient programs. Limited data comes from observational studies, including one of a PHP for adults [54], one of a PHP for youth [52], one

IOP with a mixed sample of adolescents and adults (age range: 15–47; [55]), and one IOP for adults [49]. Most of these studies were conducted in the context of the COVID-19 pandemic, which was the impetus for the transition to virtual care. The adult PHP included nine patients, all diagnosed with anorexia nervosa [54], and the youth PHP included 28 families (28 youth and 51 caregivers), all with diagnoses of anorexia nervosa [52]. The mixed-age IOP study compared a sample of patients who participated in an in-person IOP pre-pandemic ($n = 60$) to a group who partici-pated in a virtual IOP during the pandemic ($n = 33$), with diagnoses of anorexia nervosa (43%), OSFED (34%), bulimia nervosa (11%), binge-eating disorder (10%), or ARFID (2%; [55]). The adult IOP included 57 participants with diagnoses of anorexia nervosa (37%), bulimia nervosa (37%), binge-eating disorder (16%), ARFID (5%), or OSFED (5%). The programs generally transitioned all group ther-apy interventions to telehealth platforms, in addition to the family and individual therapy sessions. Some of the programs offered virtual group meal support [49, 54, 55], while the adolescent-focused program offered virtual meal support with fami-lies separately, rather than in a group format [52]. Findings were suggestive of clini-cal improvements at the end of the virtual PHP/IOP, including improvements in BMI [54, 55], eating disorder symptoms [49, 54, 55], perfectionism [55]; depres-sion [49, 54, 55], anxiety symptoms [54], self-esteem [49], and quality of life [49]. In the only study that compared outcomes to a previous cohort of the in-person IOP, patients in the virtual IOP made similar progress to participants from the in-person IOP [55].

In terms of the patient experience of the online intensive outpatient and partial hospitalization programs, adult participants rated high satisfaction with the virtual IOP [49]. In the youth-focused PHP, youth rated meal support, family sessions, and individual sessions as less helpful virtually than in person and were more likely to report a desire to return to in-person care, while parents rated virtual and in-person interventions as about equal and were open to or even preferred virtual care moving forward [52]. Some of the same benefits of telehealth described for outpatient ther-apy were also reported, such as appreciation for ease of access and increased flexi-bility with online modalities [52], and similar disadvantages were also described, such as feeling a reduced connection or alliance with other participants [52].

Though the outcomes were promising, there were some specific challenges in transitioning IOP and PHP interventions to virtual care. It is noted that facilitating groups virtually can be challenging, as conversations among group members may be less spontaneous, and there can be difficulty reading body language, interactions, and reactions among group members [54]. It is suggested that the group leader may need to take an especially active role in leading the group, including making objec-tives clear and directly inviting group members to speak by calling on them [54]. An additional strategy suggested is to ask group members to complete a therapeutic activity during the session individually and then share the product with the group and for the facilitator or participants to use the chat function as needed [54]. In many video platforms, the participant's name appears on the screen with their video image, and group leaders may suggest that participants include only their first name to protect confidentiality [49].

A component of many intensive outpatient and partial hospitalization programs is meal support. During in-person programs, this typically involves patients eating with the support of staff, with supervision to ensure meal completion and adequate caloric intake. In programs involving youth, meal support also often incorporates caregivers [52]. For individuals participating in treatment individually, the lack of in-person meal support was noted to be the most challenging aspect of the transition to virtual care, as there is no direct supervision available to ensure adequate food intake [54]. In the virtual adult programs, patients completed online meal support, where they were asked to prepare their meals at home and join the group via video to complete their meal with other patients and staff virtually. One program obtained specific information on meal content, portions, and amount consumed by asking the patient to upload a photo of their plate before and after the meal to a HIPPA-compliant application, Recovery Record [56], for the treatment team to view [49]. It is noted that patients need to actively challenge their eating disorder cognitions by eating the amount and types of foods that are necessary for recovery, and the virtual modality may be ineffective in patients who are not ready to actively seek recovery, given that it would be possible to undereat in the virtual meal support sessions [54].

Overall, the limited extant literature on eating disorder IOP and PHP interventions via telehealth suggest it is feasible to conduct these programs online, and outcome data are promising, with one study suggesting outcomes may be similar to in-person care [55]. However, sample sizes were generally small, and the existing studies were observational and primarily conducted in the context of COVID-19. Randomized controlled trials are needed to clarify how virtual intensive outpatient and partial hospitalization programs compare to their in-person counterparts. Further, each of the programs examined in these studies had different therapeutic philosophies and treatment components (e.g., CBT-based, family-based, exposure-based), and it is unclear how different treatment approaches may have impacted participant experience and progress. There were some challenges reported with the IOP and PHP levels of care that may make in-person treatment a preferred modality for patients with the acuity of illness requiring this level of care [52]. Nonetheless, this preliminary data on virtual intensive outpatient and partial hospitalization programs suggest that they may be effective and promising options that could increase treatment access for patients and families beyond the pandemic [55].

Residential and Inpatient Treatment

By definition, inpatient and residential eating disorder treatment involve 24/7 medical and/or psychiatric care for the most acutely ill patients, and thus it is not appropriate to shift to entirely virtual interventions for these levels of care. However, virtual care has been used to enhance the involvement of family members who are not able to be physically present, by attending scheduled virtual meetings with patients and staff [50]. Some residential treatment programs also offer virtual psychoeducational "family days" to provide additional psychoeducation and support to families. Additionally, in the context of the COVID-19 pandemic, some inpatient programs conducted patient groups virtually to allow staff and patients to socially distance and/or for some staff members to work off-site [50]. These creative strategies will be useful to consider beyond the pandemic, to effectively involve caregivers in a geographical location different from the treatment center.

Conclusions

Eating disorders are serious illnesses with significant medical and psychiatric impacts, and access to evidence-based care for eating disorders has historically been limited by a shortage of highly trained providers combined with geographical constraints. Telehealth interventions for eating disorders are emerging as one potential solution to increasing access [21]. Though the literature on uses of telehealth in the treatment of eating disorders remains relatively sparse, and most studies occurred in the context of the COVID-19 pandemic, many aspects of eating disorder management, especially outpatient psychotherapies, appear to be highly adaptable to telehealth interventions. Further research is needed on medical management strategies via telehealth, and larger, randomized studies of telehealth interventions for eating disorders in youth are necessary to clarify best practice guidelines.

References

1. American Psychiatric Association. (2013) Diagnostic and statistical manual of mental disorders (5th edition). https://doi.org/10.1176/appi.books.9780890425596.
2. Arcelus J, Mitchell AJ, Wales J, Nielsen S. Mortality rates in patients with anorexia nervosa and other eating disorders: a meta-analysis of 36 studies. JAMA Psychiatry. 2011;68(7):724–31. https://doi.org/10.1001/archgenpsychiatry.2011.74.
3. van Hoeken D, Hoek HW. Review of the burden of eating disorders: mortality, disability, costs, quality of life, and family burden. Curr Opin Psychiatry. 2020;33(6):521–7. https://doi.org/10.1097/YCO.0000000000000641.
4. Golden NH, Katzman DK, Sawyer SM, Society for Adolescent Health and Medicine, et al. Position paper of the Society for Adolescent Health and Medicine: medical management of restrictive eating disorders in adolescents and young adults. J Adolesc Health. 2015;56(1):121–5. https://doi.org/10.1016/j.jadohealth.2014.10.259.
5. Bulik CM, Thornton L, Pinheiro AP, Plotnicov K, Klump KL, Brandt H, Crawford S, Fichter MM, Halmi KA, Johnson C, Kaplan AS, Mitchell J, Nutzinger D, Strober M, Treasure J, Woodside DB, Berrettini WH, Kaye WH. Suicide attempts in anorexia nervosa. Psychosom Med. 2008;70(3):378–83. https://doi.org/10.1097/PSY.0b013e3181646765.
6. Franko DL, Keel PK. Suicidality in eating disorders: occurrence, correlates, and clinical implications. Clin Psychol Rev. 2006;26(6):769–82. https://doi.org/10.1016/j.cpr.2006.04.001.
7. Sansone RA, Levitt JL. Self-harm behaviors among those with eating disorders: an overview. Eat Disord. 2002;10(3):205–13. https://doi.org/10.1080/10640260290081786.
8. Yao S, Kuja-Halkola R, Thornton LM, Runfola CD, D'Onofrio BM, Almqvist C, Lichtenstein P, Sjölander A, Bulik CM. Familial liability for eating disorders and suicide attempts: evi-

dence from a population registry in Sweden. JAMA Psychiatry. 2016;73(3):284–91. https://doi.org/10.1001/jamapsychiatry.2015.2737.
9. DeLeel ML, Hughes TL, Miller JA, Hipwell A, Theodore LA. Prevalence of eating disturbance and body image dissatisfaction in young girls: an examination of the variance across racial and socioeconomic groups. Psychol Sch. 2009;46(8):767–75. https://doi.org/10.1002/pits.20415.
10. Gard MC, Freeman CP. The dismantling of a myth: a review of eating disorders and socioeconomic status. Int J Eat Disord. 1996;20(1):1–12. https://doi.org/10.1002/(SICI)1098-108X(199607)20:1<1::AID-EAT1>3.0.CO;2-M.
11. Rogers L, Resnick MD, Mitchell JE, Blum RW. The relationship between socioeconomic status and eating-disordered behaviors in a community sample of adolescent girls. Int J Eat Disord. 1997;22(1):15–23. https://doi.org/10.1002/(sici)1098-108x(199707)22:1<15::aid-eat2>3.0.co;2-5.
12. Gorrell S, Loeb KL, Le Grange D. Family-based treatment of eating disorders: a narrative review. Psychiatr Clin N Am. 2019;42(2):193–204. https://doi.org/10.1016/j.psc.2019.01.004.
13. Lock J, Le Grange D. Family-based treatment: where are we and where should we be going to improve recovery in child and adolescent eating disorders. Int J Eat Disord. 2019;52:481–7. https://doi.org/10.1002/eat.22980.
14. Dalle Grave R, Eckhardt S, Calugi S, Le Grange D. A conceptual comparison of family-based treatment and enhanced cognitive behavior therapy in the treatment of adolescents with eating disorders. J Eat Disord. 2019;7:42. https://doi.org/10.1186/s40337-019-0275-x.
15. Davis C, Ng KC, Oh JY, Baeg A, Rajasegaran K, Chew CSE. Caring for children and adolescents with eating disorders in the current coronavirus 19 pandemic: a Singapore perspective. J Adolesc Health. 2020;67(1):131–4. https://doi.org/10.1016/j.jadohealth.2020.03.037.
16. Lewis YD, Elran-Barak R, Grundman-Shem Tov R, Zubery E. The abrupt transition from face-to-face to online treatment for eating disorders: a pilot examination of patients' perspectives during the COVID-19 lockdown. J Eat Disord. 2021;9(1):31. https://doi.org/10.1186/s40337-021-00383-y.
17. Schlegl S, Maier J, Meule A, Voderholzer U. Eating disorders in times of the COVID-19 pandemic—results from an online survey of patients with anorexia nervosa. Int J Eat Disord. 2020;53(11):1791–800. https://doi.org/10.1002/eat.23374.
18. Shaw H, Robertson S, Ranceva N. What was the impact of a global pandemic (COVID-19) lockdown period on experiences within an eating disorder service? A service evaluation of the views of patients, parents/carers and staff. J Eat Disord. 2021;9(1):14. https://doi.org/10.1186/s40337-021-00368-x.
19. Spigel R, Lin JA, Milliren CE, Freizinger M, Vitagliano JA, Woods ER, Forman SF, Richmond TK. Access to care and worsening eating disorder symptomatology in youth during the COVID-19 pandemic. J Eat Disord. 2021;9(1):6. https://doi.org/10.1186/s40337-021-00421-9.
20. Termorshuizen JD, Watson HJ, Thornton LM, Borg S, Flatt RE, MacDermod CM, Harper LE, van Furth EF, Peat CM, Bulik CM. Early impact of COVID-19 on individuals with self-reported eating disorders: a survey of ~1,000 individuals in the United States and The Netherlands. Int J Eat Disord. 2020;53(11):1780–90. https://doi.org/10.1002/eat.23353.
21. Kazdin AE, Fitzsimmons-Craft EE, Wilfley DE. Addressing critical gaps in the treatment of eating disorders. Int J Eat Disord. 2017;50:170–89. https://doi.org/10.1002/eat.22670.
22. Sproch LE, Anderson KP. Clinician-delivered teletherapy for eating disorders. Psychiatr Clin N Am. 2019;42(2):243–52. https://doi.org/10.1016/j.psc.2019.01.008.
23. Barney A, Buckelew S, Mesheriakova V, Raymond-Flesch M. The COVID-10 pandemic and rapid implementation of adolescent and young adult telemedicine: challenge and opportunities for innovation. J Adolesc Health. 2020;67(2):164–71. https://doi.org/10.1016/j.jadohealth.2020.05.006.
24. Wood SM, White K, Peebles R, Pickel J, Alausa M, Mehringer J, Dowshen N. Outcomes of a rapid adolescent telehealth scale-up during the COVID-19 pandemic. J Adolesc Health. 2020;67(2):172–8. https://doi.org/10.1016/j.jadohealth.2020.05.025.

25. Couturier J, Pellegrini D, Miller C, Bhatnagar N, Boachie A, Bourret K, Brouwers M, Coelho JS, Dimitropoulos G, Findlay S, Ford C, Geller J, Grewal S, Gusella J, Isserlin L, Jericho M, Johnson N, Katzman DK, Kimber M, et al. The COVID-19 pandemic and eating disorders in children, adolescents, and emerging adults: virtual care recommendations from the Canadian consensus panel during COVID-19 and beyond. J Eat Disord. 2021b;9(1):46. https://doi.org/10.1186/s40337-021-00394-9.

26. Abrahamsson N, Ahlund L, Ahrin E, Alfonsson S. Video-based CBT-E improves eating patterns in obese patients with eating disorder: a single case multiple baseline study. J Behav Ther Exp Psychiatry. 2018;61:104–12. https://doi.org/10.1016/j.jbtep.2018.06.010.

27. Bakke B, Mitchell J, Wonderlich S, Erickson R. Administering cognitive-behavioral therapy for bulimia nervosa via telemedicine in rural settings. Int J Eat Disord. 2001;30(4):454–7. https://doi.org/10.1002/eat.1107.

28. Hamatani S, Numata N, Matsumoto K, Sutoh C, Ibuki H, Oshiro K, et al. Internet-based cognitive behavioral therapy via videoconference for patients with bulimia nervosa and binge-eating disorder: pilot prospective single-arm feasibility trial. JMIR Form Res. 2019;3:e15738. https://doi.org/10.2196/15738.

29. Simpson S, Bell L, Britton P, Mitchell D, Morrow E, Johnston AL, Brebner J. Does video therapy work? A single case series of bulimic disorders. Eur Eat Disord Rev. 2006;14(4):226–41. https://doi.org/10.1002/erv.686.

30. Simpson S, Knox J, Mitchell D, Ferguson J, Brebner J, Brebner E. A multidisciplinary approach to the treatment of eating disorders via videoconferencing in north-East Scotland. J Telemed Telecare. 2003;9(Suppl 1):S37–8. https://doi.org/10.1258/135763303322196286.

31. Giel KE, Leehr EJ, Becker S, Herzog W, Junne F, Schmidt U, Zipfel S. Relapse prevention via videoconference for anorexia nervosa—findings from the RESTART pilot study. Psychother Psychosom. 2015;84:381–3. https://doi.org/10.1159/000431044.

32. Mitchell JE, Crosby RD, Wonderlich SA, Crow S, Lancaster K, Simonich H, Swan-Kremier L, Lysne C, Myers TC. A randomized trial comparing the efficacy of cognitive-behavioral therapy for bulimia nervosa delivered via telemedicine versus face-to-face. Behav Res Ther. 2008;46:581–92. https://doi.org/10.1016/j.brat.2008.02.004.

33. Goldfield GS, Boachie A. Case report: delivery of family therapy in the treatment of anorexia nervosa using telehealth. Telemed J E Health. 2003;9(1):111–4. https://doi.org/10.1089/153056203763317729.

34. Anderson KE, Byrne CE, Crosby RD, Le Grange D. Utilizing telehealth to deliver family-based treatment for adolescent anorexia nervosa. Int J Eat Disord. 2017;50:1235–8. https://doi.org/10.1002/eat.22759.

35. Anderson KE, Byrne C, Goodyear A, Reichel R, Le Grange D. Telemedicine of family-based treatment for adolescent anorexia nervosa: a protocol of a treatment development study. J Eat Disord. 2015;3:25. https://doi.org/10.1186/s40337-015-0063-1.

36. Raykos BC, Erceg-Hurn DM, Hill J, Campbell BNC, McEvoy PM. Positive outcomes from integrating telehealth into routine clinical practice for eating disorders during COVID-19. Int J Eat Disord. 2021;54:1689–95. https://doi.org/10.1002/eat.23574.

37. Steiger H, Booij L, Crescenzi O, Oliverio S, Singer I, Thaler L, St-Hilaire A, Israel M. In-person versus virtual therapy in outpatient eating-disorder treatment: a COVID-19 inspired study. Int J Eat Disord. 2021;55:145–50. https://doi.org/10.1002/eat.23655.

38. Hellner M, Bohon C, Kolander S, Parks E. Virtually delivered family-based eating disorder treatment using an enhanced multidisciplinary care team: a case study. Clin Case Reports. 2021;9:e04173. https://doi.org/10.1002/ccr3.4173.

39. Peterson KM, Ibañez VF, Volkert VM, Zeleny JR, Engler CW, Piazza CC. Using telehealth to provide outpatient follow-up to children with avoidant/restrictive food intake disorder. J Appl Behav Anal. 2021;54:6–24. https://doi.org/10.1002/jaba.794.

40. Couturier J, Pellegrini D, Miller C, Agar P, Webb C, Anderson K, Barwick M, Dimitropoulos G, Findlay S, Kimber M, McVey G, Lock J. Adapting and adopting highly specialized pediatric eating disorder treatment to virtual care: a protocol for an implementation study

in the COVID-19 context. Implement Sci Commun. 2021a;2:38. https://doi.org/10.1186/s43058-021-00143-8.

41. Ertelt TW, Crosby RD, Marino JM, Mitchell JE, Lancaster K, Crow SJ. Therapeutic factors affecting the cognitive behavioral treatment of bulimia nervosa via telemedicine versus face-to-face delivery. Int J Eat Disord. 2011;44:687–91. https://doi.org/10.1002/eat.20874.

42. Stewart C, Konstantellou A, Kassamali F, McLaughlin N, Cutinha D, Bryant-Waugh R, Simic M, Eisler I, Baudinet J. Is this the 'new normal'? A mixed method investigation of young person, parent, and clinician experience of online eating disorder treatment during the COVID-19 pandemic. J Eat Disord. 2021;9:78. https://doi.org/10.1186/s40337-021-00429-1.

43. Vuillier L, May L, Greville-Harris M, Surman R, Moseley RL. The impact of the COVID-19 pandemic on individuals with eating disorders: the role of emotion regulation and exploration of online treatment experiences. J Eat Disord. 2021;9:10. https://doi.org/10.1186/s40337-020-00362-9.

44. Monteleone AM, Cascino G, Barone E, Carfagno M, Monteleone P. COVID-19 pandemic and eating disorders: what can we learn about psychopathology and treatment? A systemic review. Curr Psychiatry Rep. 2021;23:83. https://doi.org/10.1007/s11920021-01294-0.

45. Weissman RS, Hay P. People's lived experience with an eating disorder during the COVID-19 pandemic: a joint virtual issue of research published in leading eating disorder journals. Int J Eat Disord. 2021;55(2):155–60. https://doi.org/10.1002/eat.23653.

46. Colleluori G, Goria I, Zillanti C, Marucci S, Ragione LD. Eating disorders during COVID-19 pandemic: the experience of Italian healthcare providers. Eat Weight Disord—Studies on Anorexia, Bulimia, and Obesity. 2021;26:2787–93. https://doi.org/10.1007/s40519-021-01116-5.

47. Matheson BE, Bohon C, Lock JL. Family-based treatment via videoconference: clinical recommendations for treatment providers during COVID-19 and beyond. Int J Eat Disord. 2020;53:1142–54. https://doi.org/10.1002/eat.23326.

48. Waller G, Pugh M, Mulkens S, et al. Cognitive-behavioral therapy in the time of coronavirus: Clinician tips for working with eating disorders via telehealth when face-to-face meetings are not possible. Int J Eat Disord. 2020;53(7):1132–41. https://doi.org/10.1002/eat.23289.

49. Blalock DV, Le Grange D, Johnson C, Duffy A, Manwaring J, Tallent CN, Schneller K, Solomon AM, Mehler PS, McClanahan SF, Rienecke RD. Pilot assessment of a virtual intensive outpatient program for adults with eating disorders. Eur Eat Disord Rev. 2020;28:789–95. https://doi.org/10.1002/erv.2785.

50. Datta N, Derenne J, Sanders M, Lock JD. Telehealth transition in a comprehensive care unit for eating disorders: challenges and long-term benefits. Int J Eat Disord. 2020;53:1774–9. https://doi.org/10.1002/eat.23348.

51. Serur Y, Enoch-Levy A, Passach I, Joffe-Milstein M, Gothelf D, Stein D. Treatment of eating disorders in adolescents during the COVID-19 pandemic: a case series. J Eat Disord. 2021;9:17. https://doi.org/10.1186/s40337-021-00374-z.

52. Brothwood PL, Baudinet J, Stewart CS, Simic M. Moving online: young people and parents' experiences of adolescent eating disorder day programme treatment during the COVID-19 pandemic. J Eat Disord. 2021;9:62. https://doi.org/10.1186/s40337-021-00418-4.

53. American Psychological Association (2006) Practice Guideline for the treatment of patients with eating disorders, 3rd edition. https://psychiatryonline.org/pb/assets/raw/sitewide/practice_guidelines/guidelines/eatingdisorders.pdf

54. Plumley S, Kristensen A, Jenkins PE. Continuation of an eating disorders day programme during the COVID-19 pandemic. J Eat Disord. 2021;9:34. https://doi.org/10.1186/s40337-021-00390-z.

55. Levinson CA, Spoor SP, Keshishian AC, Pruitt A. Pilot outcomes from a multidisciplinary telehealth versus in-person intensive outpatient program for eating disorders during versus before the Covid-19 pandemic. Int J Eat Disord. 2021;54(9):1672–9. https://doi.org/10.1002/eat.23579.

56. Tregarthen JP, Lock J, Darcy AM. Development of a smartphone application for eating disorder self-monitoring. Int J Eat Disord. 2015;48:972–82. https://doi.org/10.1002/eat.22386.

Chapter 9
Adolescents and Young Adults, COVID-19, and Tele-Substance Use Treatment

Maria Rahmandar and Taraneh Shafii

The COVID-19 Public Health Emergency (PHE) declaration has changed the way in which substance use treatment is able to be provided. Outside of the PHE, federal regulations require establishing care with patients via *an in-person encounter prior to prescribing controlled substances* [1] *(telehealth.hhs.gov), including buprenorphine, which is an important medication for treatment of opioid use disorders. Some states that required face-to-face assessments prior to admission to substance use treatment programs also loosened this requirement to allow for engagement* via *telemedicine* [2] *(www.dhs.state.il.us). The pandemic precipitated policy liberation, care model expansion, and technology innovation to provide harm-reduction and life-saving care* [3]. *Without permanent revision of these regulations at a federal level, access to substance use treatment* via *telemedicine may become more limited following the end of the PHE.*

M. Rahmandar
Lurie Children's Hospital, Chicago, IL, USA
e-mail: MRahmandar@luriechildrens.org

T. Shafii (✉)
University of Washington, Seattle, WA, USA

Seattle Children's Hospital, Seattle, WA, USA
e-mail: Taraneh.shafii@seattlechildrens.org

Epidemiology of Substance Use in Adolescents and Young Adults

In a national representative sample of adolescents attending school in the USA, the prevalence of substance use remained stable in 2022 compared to the significant decrease seen the previous year. The use reduction in 2021 was deemed related to the COVID-19 pandemic with closed schools and social distancing. In 12th graders, nicotine vaping (27%) and cannabis use (31%) remained stable, while alcohol use (52%) and non-heroin narcotic use (1.7%) returned to pre-pandemic levels [4]. The overall trend of low and stable illicit drug use in adolescents is incongruent with the dramatic rise in overdose mortality and largely attributable to fentanyl fatalities which increased for 14–18-year-olds from 1 per 100,000 in 2019 to 4 per 100,000 in 2021 [5].

Accessibility and Convenience

To provide adolescents and young adults (AYA) access to treatment for substance use disorder during the COVID-19 pandemic, face-to-face visits were quickly converted to virtual appointments through telemedicine [6–8] which AYA found acceptable; however, they reported a preference for individual virtual visits over virtual group therapy [9].

In addition to the benefit of social distancing during the pandemic, telemedicine eliminated barriers that existed pre-pandemic by facilitating access for youth without transportation to or living far distances from healthcare providers.

Virtual visits also allow care continuity for youth with busy schedules who may have otherwise cancelled in-person visits due to obligations of school, work, sports, and other extracurricular activities. In qualitative studies pre- and post-pandemic, AYA echoed the convenience of easy scheduling and no travel time for virtual visits [9, 10], and post-pandemic they appreciated seeing their provider's face while remaining at a safe distance [9].

Motivation to Participate in Treatment and Potential Distractions

Attending visits from the privacy of home bedrooms also carry distractions with some youth focused more on their cell phone screen than the screen showing their provider. AYA acknowledges there are more distractions, interruptions, and challenges in focusing during virtual visits [9] as compared to face-to-face visits. The accessibility and convenience of telemedicine works best for those motivated to participate in treatment as there are reports from providers of patients listening to loud music or even silently with headphones during sessions, and some youth may even smoke or use e-cigarettes in front of the provider.

Confidentiality Pros and Cons

For some youth, interacting with providers virtually feels safer and more private than walking into a clinic. Others may have the challenge of finding a quiet space for the telemedicine session in a busy household with few private spaces. Priorities and availability of AYA differ, and providers may be surprised by the unpredictable location patients connect from virtually such as a restaurant drive-thru, outing with friends, or from their place of work, all of which have inherent interruptions and offer minimal privacy.

Rapport Building for Both Providers and Patients

While some patients may feel more secure with virtual encounters, clinicians may have difficulty establishing rapport and engaging new patients who may be in treatment reluctantly. AYA shared the same challenge of developing rapport with providers virtually. Specifically, they described telemedicine visits as less personal, difficult to read body language, and awkward to discuss sensitive issues over video [9].

Strategies to Overcome Challenges

Clinicians may be better able to continue rapport and connection virtually when the introductory visit and initial assessment were completed with the youth in person. While a patient may also be disengaged with face-to-face visits, the clinic room provides a space with fewer external distractions for the duration of the encounter, and the provider may be better skilled at in-person rapport building than virtual. If the first visit to establish care was virtual and the clinician-client connection is tenuous, one strategy is to initiate a hybrid model of intermittent in-person visits incorporated within the virtual model of care or if that is insufficient then move to all in-person visits for the remainder of treatment.

Innovation to Increase Family Involvement

The COVID pandemic fueled innovation in conceptual frameworks to accommodate treatment needs. While some youth may prefer not to have family involved in substance use treatment and are legally entitled to confidential care in most states, telemedicine lends well to family involvement. A conceptual framework was developed to enhance telemedicine interventions in the treatment of opioid use disorders in youth through family outreach, engagement, training, and recovery maintenance [11]. The model has yet to be tested for efficacy but has succeeded in increasing family accessibility to care and in reducing logistic barriers (e.g., work absence, childcare, transportation, and cost) to participating in their child's treatment [12]. Pre-COVID, in a qualitative analysis, online counseling via real-time web chat for those (mostly adults and less than 30% AYA) using substances and their family and friends enabled accessibility to services, distress tolerance, action planning, and enhanced communication [13].

Acceptability and Efficacy Studies

Work to explore the usefulness of telemedicine to treat substance use in youth had already begun pre-pandemic. Telemedicine for SUD prevention and HIV risk reduction was found to be feasible and acceptable in a pilot study of rural African American adolescents [14] and HIV-positive young adults [15]. AYA are accepting of telemedicine, and it has been found to be as effective or more so than face-to-face visits in the treatment of substance use disorders. In a recent review of studies conducted pre-pandemic, virtual motivational interviewing and videoconferencing were found effective in AYA for reducing alcohol and tobacco use [16–18]. In a randomized controlled trial of college students who binge drink, the intervention was delivered using videoconference or face-to-face, and both modalities were equally effective in reducing alcohol use [19]. In addition, in a longitudinal study of intensive outpatient treatment for addiction, no differences were found in continuous abstinence with in-person, hybrid, or virtual care models. Of note, most of this later study population were adults with AYA comprising 12% of the study sample and outcomes were not stratified by age [7].

Conclusion

Out of necessity, the COVID-19 pandemic accelerated innovation in models for substance use treatment. Telemedicine visits are acceptable to and feasible in adolescents and young adults. Many logistical barriers in accessing care are eliminated, and yet this convenience needs to be balanced with potential difficulties in developing rapport with new patients and the increased distractions for patients attending visits from their bedrooms. Efficacy studies to date show promise that telemedicine visits provide the same if not better outcomes in the treatment of substance use disorder. To ensure the highest-risk patients receive life-saving care, it is important for telemedicine to remain a treatment option in the post-pandemic era.

Case 1: Engaged Patient with Issues Accessing Care in Person

An 18-year-old female who was referred to substance use treatment by her primary care provider. She was primarily interested in addressing her cocaine use. She attends school several hours from clinic. With telemedicine, she was able to engage in treatment with a substance use program and start cutting back and eventually stop her cocaine use. However, since she was not attending the program in person, she did not initially or routinely provide urine drug tests, which limited the therapist's ability to objectively monitor for recurrence of cocaine use and prevented the therapist from assessing urine for fentanyl adulteration of the patient's cocaine supply. Eventually, the patient was able to attend the program in person where urine testing was completed after a recent recurrence of cocaine use, no fentanyl was identified on send-out testing, and the patient was given several fentanyl test strip kits to be able to test her drug supply in case she used cocaine again. However, with continued engagement via telemedicine, she was able to stop cocaine use and continues to work on nicotine use.

Key Points to Consider:

- Telemedicine helps with accessibility to care and treatment programs, especially in motivated patients.
- Inability to provide urine drug screens (UDS) should not prevent engagement in treatment. Monitor behaviors, not just UDS.
- When drug screens can be helpful, consider random calls to send to outside labs or using home testing protocols, where a family obtains urine cups from a local lab and ideally obtains first morning urine (where urine is most concentrated) that is returned to the lab. Home testing should be done in collaboration with a medical provider, as parent-led testing using commercially available home tests can lead to misinterpretation and potentially further strain the parent-child relationship [20] (AAP).

Case 2: Out of State Telemedicine and Issues with Prescription Medications

A 17-year-old female was referred to substance use treatment after being seen in the emergency department following several episodes of sex trafficking. After many recurrences of opioid and other substance use, she needed a change in environment, attended residential treatment, and subsequently moved out of state to live with other supportive family members. Through flexibilities in telemedicine regulations during the public health emergency (PHE), she was able to continue to re-engage with previous treatment providers via telemedicine, though they were out of state. However, restrictions around out-of-state controlled substance prescriptions prevented her from being able to continue to receive her life-saving medication for opioid use disorder, buprenorphine. She had to travel back to her previous state to obtain her prescriptions.

Key Points to Consider

- Telemedicine flexibilities during the PHE helped with access to care but differing state, hospital, and pharmacy regulations and restrictions around controlled substance prescriptions limit care. Providers can advocate for changes to these regulations, but until they are changed, providers may be able to prescribe to pharmacies along state borders that may be more accessible to patients out-of-state, obtain medical licenses in surrounding states, or collaborate with local care providers, including primary care providers, to help build local capacity to provide medication for addiction treatment.

Case 3: Adolescent Logs in from Public Spaces and Uses Drugs During Their Appointment

A 16-year-old male has been engaged in therapy for marijuana and alcohol use. He often asks to change in-person appointments to telemedicine when he has work or school. Sometimes, he will be on the bus or other public spaces during appointments. Occasionally, he is noted to be vaping during sessions with provider.

Key Points to Consider:

- Though telemedicine offers flexibility in location of patient, certain spaces may not be conducive to honest discussion of sensitive subjects.
- Telemedicine offers opportunities to continue to connect with patients reluctantly in treatment when they might otherwise have cancelled.
- It is a delicate balance for providers to witness the very behaviors which they are trying to change while maintaining rapport and patient engagement.

Acknowledgments Kelly Kerby CDMHP for clinical experience, insights, and perspective.

References

1. Prescribing controlled substances via telehealth. https://telehealth.hhs.gov/providers/policy-changes-during-the-covid-19-public-health-emergency/prescribing-controlled-substances-via-telehealth/. Accessed 16 Dec 2022.
2. 3/16/20-Message to substance use prevention & recovery providers—COVID-19 Frequently Asked Questions. https://www.dhs.state.il.us/page.aspx?item=123262. Accessed 15 Dec 2022.
3. Krawczyk N, Fawloe A, Yang J, Tofighi B. Early innovations in opioid use disorder treatment and harm reduction during the COVID-19 pandemic: a scoping review. Addict Sci Clin Pract. 2021;16(68):1–15.
4. NIDA. Most reported substance use among adolescents held steady in 2022. National Institute on Drug Abuse website. https://nida.nih.gov/news-events/news-releases/2022/12/most-reported-substance-use-among-adolescents-held-steady-in-2022. Accessed 16 Dec 2022.
5. Friedman J, Godvin M, Shover CL, Gone JP, Hansen H, Schriger DL. Trends in drug overdose deaths among US adolescents, January 2010 to June 2021. JAMA. 2022;327(14):1398–400. https://doi.org/10.1001/jama.2022.2847.
6. Komaromy M, Tomanovich M, Taylor J, Ruiz-Mercado G, Kimmel S, Bagley S. Adaptation of a system of treatment for substance use disorders during the COVID-19 pandemic. J Addict Med. 2021;15(6):448–51.
7. Gliske K, Welsh J, Braughton J, Walsh NQ. Telehealth services for substance use disorders during the COVID-19 pandemic: longitudinal assessment of intensive outpatient programming and data collection practices. JMIR Ment Health. 2022;9(3):1–12.
8. Langabeer J, Yatsco A, Champagne-Langabeer T. Telehealth sustains patient engagement in OUD treatment during COVID-19. J Subst Abus Treat. 2021;122:1–3.
9. Hawke L, Sheikhan N, MacCon K, Henderson J. Going virtual: youth attitudes toward and experience of virtual mental health and substance use services during the COVID-19 pandemic. BMC Health Serv Res. 2021;21(340):1–10.
10. Saberi P, Rose C, Wootton A, Ming K, Legnitto D, Jeske M, et al. Use of technology for delivery of mental health and substance use services to youth living with HIV: a mixed methods perspective. AIDS Care. 2020;32(8):931–9.
11. Hogue A, Bobek M, Levy S, Henderson C, Fishman M, Becker S, et al. Conceptual framework for telehealth strategies to increase family involvement in treatment and recovery for youth opioid use disorder. J Marital Fam Ther. 2021;47:501–14.

12. Hogue A, Becker S, Fishman M, Henderson C, Levy S. Youth OUD treatment during and after COVID: increasing family involvement across the services continuum. J Subst Abuse Treat. 2021;120:1–3.
13. Dilkes-Frayne E, Savic M, Carter A, Kokanovic R, Lubman D. Going online: the affordances of online counseling for families affected by alcohol and other drug issues. Qual Health Res. 2019;29(14):2010–22.
14. Lopez C, Gilmore A, Moreland A, Danielson C, Acierno R. Meeting kids where they are at—a substance use and sexual risk prevention program via telemedicine for African American girls: usability and acceptability study. J Med Internet Res. 2020;22(8):1–14.
15. Saberi P, McCuistian C, Agnew E, Wootton A, Packard D, Dawson-Rose C. Video-counseling intervention to address HIV care engagement, mental health, and substance use challenges: a pilot randomized clinical trial for youth and young adults living with HIV. Telemed Rep. 2021;2(1):14–23.
16. Byaruhanga J, Atorkey P, McLaughlin M, Brown A, Byrnes E, Paul C, et al. Effectiveness of individual real-time video counseling on smoking, nutrition, alcohol, physical activity, and obesity health risk: systematic review. J Med Internet Res. 2020;22(9):1–17.
17. Kruse C, Lee K, Watson H, Lobo L, Stoppelmoor A, Oyibo A. Measures of effectiveness, efficiency, and quality of telemedicine in the management of alcohol abuse, addiction, and rehabilitation: systematic review. J Med Internet Res. 2020;22(1):1–8.
18. Caballeria E, Lopez-Pelayo H, Matrai S, Gual A. Telemedicine in the treatment of addictions. Curr Opin Psychiatry. 2022;35:227–36.
19. King S, Richner K, Tuliao A, Kennedy J, McChargue D. A comparison between telehealth and face-to-face delivery of a brief alcohol intervention for college students. Subst Abus. 2020;41(4):501–9.
20. Levy S, Siqueira L. Committee on Substance Clinical Report: testing for drugs of abuse in children and adolescents. https://publications.aap.org/pediatrics/article/133/6/e20140865/76085/Testing-for-Drugs-of-Abuse-in-Children-and-Adolescents. Accessed 16 Dec 2022.

Chapter 10
Adolescent Depression and Anxiety and the Use of Telemedicine Services to Improve Outcomes

Jeffery P. Greene

Abbreviations

COVID-19   Coronavirus disease of 2019
GAD-7   Generalized Anxiety Disorder 7
PHQ-9   Patient Health Questionnaire 9
SSRIs   Selective serotonin reuptake inhibitors

Case 1

- *A 16-year-old cisgender male presents for his annual physical exam. He is generally healthy and is not taking any medication.*
- *His mother brings up a concern that her son has had more anger outbursts.*
- *He has lost interest in sports and recently quit the high school basketball team.*
- *He spends more time alone in his bedroom on social media.*
- *GAD7 is 9/21, PHQ9 is 21/27, with a response of 2 on question #9 (thoughts being better off dead or hurting yourself in some way).*
- *He has begun giving away his most precious items to strangers.*
- *He recently ended a relationship with his girlfriend, whom he had planned to go to college with.*
- *He is unsure of what he is going to do after he graduates from high school now.*
- *Mom wants to know if he might be dealing with depression.*

J. P. Greene (✉)
University of Washington, Seattle, WA, USA

Seattle Children's Hospital, Seattle, WA, USA
e-mail: jeffery.greene@seattle.childrens.org

© The Author(s), under exclusive license to Springer Nature Switzerland AG 2024
Y. N. Evans et al. (eds.), *Telemedicine for Adolescent and Young Adult Health Care*, https://doi.org/10.1007/978-3-031-55760-6_10

Introduction

Awareness of adolescent mental health conditions, including depression and anxiety, has been brought to the forefront and is now considered its own epidemic. The Centers for Disease Control and Prevention (CDC) reports that 9.4% children and teens up to 17 years old have been diagnosed with anxiety, while 4.4% have clinical depression between 2016 and 2019 [1]. More recently, a surge of mental health conditions among teens and young adults has overwhelmed a health-care system that has been challenged to meet their demands in a timely manner. Psychiatric experts have provided practice guidelines for primary care providers, in collaboration with a multidisciplinary team, to identify and initiate treatment, and recommend that all teenagers be screened for depression and anxiety annually [2]. Time and awareness are critical, in regard to suicide prevention, as teens with depression are at a high risk for poor outcomes during the month prior to seeking medical attention. Additionally, a high number of adolescents who have died by suicide were seen by their medical provider within the previous 3 months [3].

During the COVID pandemic, social separation from peers and classmates contributing to the exacerbation of depression and anxiety risks further increased awareness and led to the epidemic reference. Teens, during a critical time of psychosocial development, and college-aged students, who were preparing themselves for their first time away from home, were quickly transitioned to remote learning. Though the immediate effects may have been a positive experience for some, over time the uncertain future, loss of control, and elimination of physical connections all had negative consequences, leading to increased depression and suicidal thinking [4–7].

Transition to virtual learning to prevent further transmission of COVID-19 resulted in social isolation and an increase incidence of depression and anxiety. Contingency plans were adopted to maintain medical readiness and operational capabilities while protecting the health and safety of frontline providers. Telehealth has become a novel concept along the primary care service line that has not only improved access for patients to readily address their health needs but also improved overall satisfaction among patient and families, as well as medical providers [8, 9]. Telehealth also addresses the health disparities that has inherently had a negative effect on health-care outcomes. One study showed the improvement in attendance when transitioning from in-person visits to virtual appointments [10]. This improved access to care also affords the opportunity to comply with the federal guidelines, regarding follow-up care for teens and young adults diagnosed with major depressive disorder and prescribed antidepressants [11].

Serotonin reuptake inhibitors (SSRIs) are the most common antidepressants prescribed to adolescents and young adults. These medications are safe and effective and decrease suicidal behaviors when started expeditiously and with caution. However, the 2004 Black Box Warning, indicating risk for increased suicidal ideations when starting SSRIs led to prescriber hesitancy, resulting in increased completed suicide when treatment was withheld [12].

SSRIs have historically demonstrated a positive effect in reducing suicidal behaviors. Furthermore, psychiatrists have adopted guidelines to reduce medication adverse reactions so psychopharmaceuticals can be swiftly prescribed while maintaining the highest level of safety, thus reducing potential for harm [2].

Major Depressive Disorder

When making a diagnosis of major depressive disorder, providers must consider the number of episodes that have occurred without evidence of mania or hypomania or other explanations for the depressive symptoms, such as substance abuse or endocrine dysfunction [13]. There must be at least five key symptoms that have occurred over a period of at least 2 weeks. Using the PHQ-9A for screening of adolescents for depression has been validated and is recommended annually [11, 14]. The revised questionnaire includes irritable mood since it is common for teenagers to experience anger problems or increased irritability rather than sadness as a symptom of depression:

Mood: anhedonia or irritability.
Sleep: insomnia or hypersomnia.
Interests: diminished interest in activities that normally bring enjoyment.
Guilt: a sense of self-worthlessness.
Energy: energy level is decreased.
Concentration: decreased concentration or ability to think.
Appetite: appetite is either diminished or increased, "comfort eating" measures.
Psychomotor features: psychomotor restriction (slowness) or agitation (restlessness).
Suicidality: increased suicidal ideation, with or without intent, specific planning or previous history of suicidal attempts.

Management of depression depends on the severity of the condition, as medication is reserved for more severe cases. Mild depression can be followed up by the primary care provider while considering a referral for cognitive behavior therapy (CBT). Additionally, duration of symptoms should also be weighed, as more mild symptoms for greater than 1 year (dysthymia) may warrant psychopharmacology consideration. For more successful outcomes when treating moderate to severe depression in teens, combination therapy (medication + CBT) has been shown to be more effective (73%) when compared to medication alone (62%) or CBT alone, which resulted in improvement in 48% of cases [15]. While an inherent risk for increased suicidal thinking exists when introducing medication to treat depression, these behaviors are reduced when combined with CBT [15].

Who Is at Risk for Suicide?

Suicide is the leading cause of death among adolescents, now being recognized as the second most common reason [16]. While females attempt suicide more commonly, death by suicide is more likely among males due to their more lethal method of choice [16]. Suicide risk assessment is of the utmost importance when evaluating teens who have been diagnosed with major depressive disorder. Other factors to consider when evaluating an adolescent for suicide risk include previous history of suicide attempt, family history of mental health conditions and suicidal behaviors, substance use, personal diagnosis of bipolar disorder, history of trauma or abuse, or self-identifying as transgender [16]. Internet use has become a social norm, but access to violent images and social media platforms, as well as duration of time spent connected to the internet, is directly correlated with increased depressed mood and suicidality among children and adolescents [16, 17]. In addition, being a victim of cyberbullying is a predictive factor for future suicidal behaviors [16]. Adolescents may present to their primary care clinic with physical symptoms, poor sleep, declining school performance, eating disorders, or other complaints that may not be recognized as depression and therefore potentially delaying diagnosis and treatment, placing the teen at risk for completed suicide.

When interviewing an adolescent, assessing for suicide risk should become part of daily practice since teens, parents, school officials, or health-care providers may not associate trivial symptoms with depression or suicide thinking. Many health organizations have included brief suicide risk assessments into the daily routine. For instance, the Ask Suicide-Screening Questions (ASQ) is a series of questions with "yes" or "no" responses that inquire about past and recent suicidal thinking [3]. In addition, the teen is asked if they are currently feeling suicidal. Depending on the number of "yes" responses, immediate referral to a mental health specialist may be necessary, especially if the teen is having current thoughts of death and suicide. However, not all patients will require this additional assessment. Subsequent to the ASQ, a primary care provider or mental health specialist may use the Brief Suicide Safety Assessment (BSSA), which offers the clinician the opportunity to assist the teen with the development of strategies to lower the risk of self-harm and suicide [3]. Since suicide is not considered protected under the laws of confidentiality, the BSSA also addresses parental awareness of the suicide risk, previous measures taken to keep the teen safe (removing access to medication, removal of kitchenware or weapons), and actions to take if the teen becomes suicidal.

In the first case, the teenager was diagnosed with major depressive disorder and immediately referred to the behavioral health team for suicide assessment. He was started on medication (Table 10.1), referred for long-term therapy, and encouraged to follow up within the first 2 weeks of initiating treatment.

Table 10.1 Selective serotonin reuptake inhibitors to treat anxiety and depression in teens (adapted from Stahl's essential psychopharmacology Prescriber's Guide, children and adolescents)

Medication	Diagnosis	Starting dose	Dose titration	Max dose	Side effects
Fluoxetine	Depression, OCD	10 mg	10 mg every 2–4 weeks	60–80 mg; >40 may not be effective for depression	Insomnia, anxiety, sexual dysfunction, longer half-life: 6–7 days
Sertraline	Depression, GAD, OCD, PTSD	25 mg	25–50 mg every 2–4 weeks	200 mg	GI: Dyspepsia, abdominal pain, diarrhea
Escitalopram	Depression, anxiety, or panic attacks	5 mg	5 mg every 1–2 weeks	20 mg	Prolonged QT interval > 20 mg

Case 2

- *A 10-year-old cisgender female with chronic recurrent abdominal pain presents with an acute recurrence of the pain over a period of 1 month.*
- *Pain is periumbilical and does not radiate. Pain is triggered by stress and unrelieved after defecation.*
- *She is a survivor of a sexual assault 1 year prior, resulting in anxiety symptoms that have required trauma therapy. She had been previously diagnosed with major depressive disorder (MDD) and post-traumatic stress disorder (PTSD).*
- *Abdominal pain has caused frequent school absenteeism and mom has left the workforce to care for child at home.*
- *Trauma therapy has reduced child's fears and she began transitioning back to in-person learning. However, mom's return to work triggered more anxiety and recurrence of the abdominal pain.*
- *She would excessively cry whenever separated from her mother, causing regression and refusal to go to school.*
- *Sleep was not disturbed and abdominal pain, though still present, was less dysfunctional on the weekends.*
- *There is a family history of depression in both mother and older brother, who both have been prescribed fluoxetine.*

Anxiety Disorder

Anxiety is the most common mental health disorder among children and adolescents and has increased in prevalence over time, ranging from 8% to 31% [18–20]. Females are affected twice as often as males, and anxiety may start at any time during childhood [19]. However, anxiety may not cause dysfunction until after entering school. Mild symptoms may cause little impairment, and therefore treatment is not considered. In more severe cases, especially if left untreated, anxiety may lead to other mental health conditions or substance use disorders as an approach to lessen the symptoms of anxiety [18, 19]. Teenagers may present with common somatic complaints, including headaches, abdominal pain, and poor sleep, ultimately diagnosed with anxiety after careful evaluation for organic causes [18, 19].

There are multiple forms of anxiety that a provider may encounter, each occurring at different ages (Table 10.2). Though each entity may have its own uniqueness, these anxiety conditions also share similarities: excessive fear exceeding what is considered normal, avoidance of a stressor that incites the fear, and excessive worrying over the anticipation of engagement with a triggering event [20].

During adolescence, the most used screening tool to assess for anxiety is the Generalized Anxiety Disorder-7 (GAD-7) questionnaire. The GAD-7 is a 7-item survey, based on the diagnostic criteria of GAD, utilized to measure severity of symptoms related to anxiety, with a score less than 5 being a negative screen. Mild symptoms of anxiety would generate a score of 5–9; moderate symptoms, 10–14; and severe symptoms, 15–21 [21]. The GAD-7 (and the PHQ-9) is validated for adolescents aged 12 and older, with the higher reliability for anxiety, the higher the score, particularly when greater than 10 [21]. Though these tools are quick and very useful in a clinical setting, they do not replace the importance of making a sound clinical decision to support the results of the screening instrument while ruling out organic causes for any symptoms that may also be associated with anxiety.

The patient in Case 2 was diagnosed with anxiety disorder, along with the prior diagnoses of major depressive disorder (MDD) and post-traumatic stress disorder (PTSD). The first-line treatment for anxiety disorder is psychotherapy. While cognitive behavioral therapy (CBT) has shown effectiveness in reducing the fear responses triggered by the anxiety-provoking stressors, medication should be considered for

Table 10.2 From diagnostic and statistical manual of mental disorders, fifth edition

Diagnosis	Associated symptoms to meet criteria
1. Generalized anxiety disorder (GAD)	Excessive worry that is difficult to control, causing changes in ability to think, sleep problems, and irritable mood, occurring for at least 6 months
2. Social anxiety	Excessive worry about being judged in social situations; avoidance of social events due to fear of rejection; anxiety is out of proportion to the level of severity of the specific triggers
3. Separation anxiety	Intense and exaggerated worry about losing relationship with a significant other, therefore refusing to leave home or to go to school
4. Panic attacks	Abrupt onset of physical symptoms (palpitations, sweating, hyperventilation, paresthesias) in response to fearful event, not explained by other mental health disorders or substance abuse disorders
5. Post-traumatic stress disorder (PTSD)	Exposure to a traumatic event (injury, sexual assault), causing recurring nightmares or flashbacks, avoidance of triggers for the traumatic event, and intense reactions, including anxiety and detachment from others
6. Obsessive-compulsive disorder (OCD)	Persistent thoughts or urges that cause significant distress, leading to repetitive behaviors in response to obsessive thoughts to reduce the anxiety experienced

those dealing with anxiety and are functionally impaired because of it. Though medications are reserved for more moderate to severe cases or when anxiety is associated with other mental health conditions, whenever there is refusal to seek therapy, medical treatment is a reasonable option, regardless of severity [18]. Escitalopram is a preferred SSRI for adolescents with generalized anxiety disorder or panic attacks [22]. Sertraline can be used for anxiety and is also approved for treatment of PTSD or OCD in childhood [22]. Fluoxetine is the most common SSRI prescribed for depression in children and adolescents and has demonstrated its safety and efficacy, particularly in teens who are dealing with hypersomnolence and psychomotor restrictions.

When considering the best option to treat depression or anxiety in adolescents, providers should consider family history and what medications have worked for first-degree relatives. Choosing the SSRI that will be most effective is a trial-and-error approach. However, it has been demonstrated that there may be a similar response to treatment among family members [23]. Though this observation has not been consistently reproduced, it is reasonable to infer that one medication that has shown benefits among first-degree relatives will also be effective for others with a familial similarity.

As previously indicated, escitalopram and sertraline are beneficial options for anxiety. However, given the age of the patient in Case 2, family history for depression, and familial response to treatment, she was started on fluoxetine. Fluoxetine is the first-line choice for adolescent depression, with a starting dose of 10–20 mg and an upper limit dose of 60–80 mg. Fluoxetine is good for teens dealing with low energy, hypersomnolence, or psychomotor restrictions. Because of its activating effects, fluoxetine is best taken in the morning, as it has been associated with insomnia. Titrating to higher doses may trigger more anxiety symptoms and agitation. Fluoxetine has a very long half-life, up to 6–7 days, and is well tolerated. For this reason, fluoxetine may be discontinued abruptly (self-weaning) if cross-titration (switching to another medication) is necessary. Weaning would be more appropriate when a patient's depressive symptoms are in remission and a decision is made by the patient and provider to discontinue treatment. Treatment of depression requires dosages between 20 and 40 mg, and doses above 40 mg are not likely to be as effective [24]. However, higher doses (60–80 mg) may be required to treat purging behaviors related to bulimia nervosa. Because of its activating effects, close monitoring for increased suicidal thoughts or any emergence of manic symptoms is imperative.

Case 3

- *A 17-year-old cisgender female with anxiety for years, usually triggered by school experiences. She is involved in extracurricular activities but has panic attacks that are provoked by start of school, exams, and family relationships.*

- *She is a high performer academically and she has a good relationship with her friends. She has a boyfriend with whom she is sexually active, and she is currently on a combined oral contraceptive pill. LMP was 2 weeks ago.*
- *GAD7 is 18/21, PHQ9 is 8/27.*
- *She worries excessively at night, causing her to lose sleep, which increases chances of having a panic attack at school. Cutting helps reduce the anxiety.*
- *She has been receiving CBT for years and wonders if medication would be helpful to calm her nerves.*
- *She has somatic complaints, including abdominal pain and headaches, that she thinks are related to her anxiety.*
- *Labs: normal CBC, CMP, TSH, vitamin D, ferritin, negative HCG.*
- *Prescribed sertraline 25 mg for 1 week, increased to 50 mg.*
- *Was instructed to follow up in 2 weeks.*
- *Returned with more pressured speech/very talkative.*
- *Worsening ability to sleep at night.*
- *Increased activities.*
- *Anxiety.*
- *No increase in suicidal thoughts.*
- *No family history of bipolar disorder.*

Assessment for adverse drug reactions is paramount when prescribing SSRIs to teenagers for depression or anxiety. When deciding to initiate therapy, it is important to start low and titrate to the therapeutic dose slowly to avoid potential, more serious side effects, including increased suicidal thoughts and treatment-emergent activation syndrome (TEAS) or hypomanic reactions [22]. Additionally, it is imperative to screen for symptoms concerning for bipolar disorder prior to starting treatment, including review of family history, as SSRIs may unmask the manic symptoms, leading to a modification of diagnosis. TEAS is a known adverse reaction caused by SSRIs, more likely to occur in medications with more activating properties. More concerning, increased activation is associated with suicidality. However, consideration should be taken that discontinuation of medication due to adverse reactions may place the adolescent at even greater risk of suicide [12, 25]. Fluoxetine, while being the most commonly prescribed of the SSRIs, is considered to be the most activating compared to other SSRIs [25]. Bupropion, a selective norepinephrine reuptake inhibitor (SNRI), a second-line treatment for adolescent depression, is another known activating medication commonly prescribed to teenagers for depression that may cause agitation and irritability [26]. The potential for the development of adverse reactions early on during medical management is the primary reason for close follow-up after treatment initiation. Prior counseling and anticipatory guidance of risks related to treatment and early recognition of medication reactions will help limit risk for self-discontinuation of therapy, which may be more ominous.

Making the decision to modify treatment based on the patient's adverse reactions requires an understanding of the treatment options, including other SSRIs, and their differing activating properties or other side effects. There are options to consider when a patient is experiencing adverse reasons, such as increased agitation, insomnia, or hyperexcitability. The risk for medication-induced activation is directly proportional to the dose of medication prescribed: the higher the dose, the more likely it is for the emergence of activating symptoms, including increased suicidality. Lowering doses of the current medication may reduce any observed side effects. However, by doing so, there is risk of lowering the therapeutic benefits of the medication. Therefore, switching to another SSRI may be a more suitable course of action to decrease the activating effects while, at the same time, reaching therapeutic potential. Though some SSRIs are more activating than others, monitoring for TEAS with any SSRI will be necessary.

For this patient in Case 3, the sertraline was discontinued abruptly since the dose was relatively low and she had been on treatment for only 2 weeks. The hypomanic symptoms resolved quickly, and given the lack of family history of bipolar disorder, the patient was ultimately diagnosed with TEAS, along with the previously diagnosed anxiety disorder. A less activating SSRI (escitalopram) was started to treat the anxiety, which did not cause a relapse of the hypomanic symptoms. The dose was titrated to effect and the anxiety symptoms subsided such that she was able to enjoy school and interact with family members more positively.

Integrating Telemedicine in the Primary Care Setting

Adolescent medicine encompasses confidential health care that includes contraceptive care, diagnosis and treatment of sexually transmitted infections, drug counseling, and mental health care. Unawareness of the rules of engagement in this setting is an unforeseen barrier to access to care. Other barriers that prevent a smooth avenue of approach when engaging the health-care system include lack of transportation and inconvenient times when teenagers prefer appointments during afterschool hours. School health clinics have opened throughout the nation to address the health disparities that place children and adolescents at risk of complications related to uncontrolled chronic illnesses that result in frequent school absenteeism and poor academic performance [27]. However, more complex conditions may require specialty care that is not readily available in the school setting.

Psychiatrists have long been able to implement telehealth services that have been accepted by patients who may have had initial concerns addressing their mental health needs through web-based media [8]. Furthermore, COVID-19 pandemic afforded opportunities to incorporate telehealth practices within the primary care medical home; barriers of care were addressed and ease of using telehealth services made it a very practical medium to connect with health-care providers [10]. The importance of close monitoring makes telehealth a feasible platform for quick assessment of response to treatment and review of any side effects. Though therapy sessions through telehealth services were not favorable, psychiatric evaluation and medication management were adaptable practices, especially during isolation caused by the COVID-19 pandemic [8, 9]. Benefits need to be weighed against the risks of using this method. While ease of delivery of services and patient preferences are critical, consideration should be taken to review actions to make when patients experience any adverse reactions to medications, especially increased suicidal thoughts. Though it is authorized to deliver confidential services, including mental health care, to minor teens (age rules vary by state), it is imperative to make it a priority to facilitate the integration of primary care givers, including parents or legal guardians, to the treatment team. Reviewing a concrete safety plan in cases where an adolescent may express suicidal thoughts is a critical piece in virtual health, where health-care professionals lose the ability to physically control a more potentially, life-threatening situation [28].

Case 4

- *A 14-year-old cisgender female who has been treated for depression with sertraline.*
- *She is adopted and lives in a safe home with adoptive parents and biological sibling, who also has significant mental conditions.*
- *She was referred to adolescent medicine due to treatment failure and evaluation took place* via *telemedicine after obtaining verbal consent.*
- *Adoptive parent was integrated into services due to teen's prior history of cutting and suicidal thoughts.*
- *She experiences significant anxiety with panic attacks, triggered by school, and prefers virtual learning and seemed to thrive during the lockdown caused by the COVID-19 pandemic.*
- *Upon return to in-person learning, the panic attacks increased despite being on the SSRI.*
- *The panic attacks triggered more non-suicidal, self-injurious behaviors, including cutting.*
- *She is currently taking sertraline 100 mg with no improvement of symptoms after 1 month on current dose. A trial of increase in dose to 150 mg yielded an increase in agitation and anxiety.*
- *Agitation lessened with lowering to prior dose; however, there was neither improvement of the overall anxiety nor her depressive symptoms.*

Sertraline is a good option for the treatment GAD, MDD, and PTSD and has been approved for the treatment of OCD in pediatric-aged patients [22]. The usual starting dose is 25 mg/day, with a therapeutic dose range of 50–200 mg. Though it usually can take 4–6 weeks to achieve adequate antidepressant effects, it is not uncommon to observe anxiolysis during the first week of treatment when targeting anxiety symptoms. Dose titration should be considered every 2–4 weeks, increasing in 25–50 mg increments to a maximum dose of 200 mg/day. Interestingly, sertraline causes more GI side effects, including nausea, dyspepsia, abdominal pain, and diarrhea compared to other SSRIs [22].

Patients will not always respond to the first antidepressant that is prescribed, so providers need to be prepared to assess the treatment goals. Further discussion with the patient whether the medication is helpful and whether any additional increase in dose of current medication will have any benefit is warranted. It is useful to consider changing to another SSRI in these cases to achieve therapeutic benefit when the first option has been exhausted. However, there is risk to changing medications, including worsening of symptoms related to the underlying condition being treated. Therefore, the benefits of the method utilized to switch to another SSRI need to be weighed against the risk for any adverse reactions [29]:

1. *Stop the first medication and immediately start the next medication at an equivalent dose (risk for withdrawal symptoms).*
2. *Taper dose until discontinuation, followed by washout period (half-life of the drug), then start new medication (risk for relapse).*
3. *Reduce current medication by 50% every 3 days until lowest dose, while starting new medication at its lowest dose and titrate to effective dose (cross-titration).*

Stopping antidepressants suddenly may risk developing withdrawal symptoms that can be intolerable, but are self-limiting [30].

FINISH *Mnemonic for Discontinuation Syndrome*

- *Flu-like symptoms, including achy muscles and chills.*
- *Insomnia or vivid dreams.*
- *Nausea.*
- *Imbalance or dizziness.*
- *Shock sensations.*
- *Hyperarousal (anxiety/agitation).*

It is vitally important to discuss the dangers of self-discontinuation of antidepressants. Informed consent and discussion of potential side effects and withdrawal symptoms prior to initiating therapy may improve compliance and treatment outcomes. Opting for medications with longer half-lives (fluoxetine) can avoid some of the negative effects caused by abrupt cessation. However, though less likely compared to other SSRIs, if side effects during treatment with fluoxetine occur and are intolerable, a patient may continue to experience these side effects for days to weeks after stopping the offending agent.

Serotonin syndrome is a potential serious consequence when taking SSRIs, especially after intentional overdose. Providers should also be aware of this reaction while changing to another SSRI where a patient may be taking two different SSRIs at the same time. A triad of symptoms that might suggest serotonin syndrome include changes in mentation (agitation, restlessness), abnormalities of neuromuscular function (hyperreflexia, tremors), and hyperactivity of the autonomic nervous system, including fever, changes in vital signs, and dilated pupils [31].

Given the activating symptoms at higher doses and lack of improvement of anxiety at current dose of sertraline in the vignette, the medication was cross-titrated with escitalopram, an approved SSRI for the treatment of anxiety and panic attacks in children and adolescents [24]:

- *Teen is taking 100 mg of sertraline- > reduced to 50 mg daily x 3 days, then 25 mg daily × 3 days.*
- *Started on escitalopram 5 mg (at the beginning of the sertraline wean) daily for 1 week and then increased to 10 mg daily.*

At the 2-week follow-up, the patient stated that she was sleeping better, had less anxiety, and was experiencing fewer panic attacks while attending class in-person.

While it is well understood that diagnosis and treatment of anxiety and depression at the primary care level should be incorporated into daily practice, how care is best delivered is a factor that requires additional investigation. Uncontrolled circumstances caused immediate adaptation to other approaches to provide needed care without interruption. Data has shown that telehealth is a desirable option for patients with mental health conditions, specifically when addressing medication management. Offering a more feasible platform to receive such services may encourage improved compliance and continuity while offering a safe and immediate bridge to address health concerns, including responses to treatment and potential adverse reactions.

References

1. Bitsko RH, Claussen AH, Lichtstein J, Black LJ, Everett Jones S, Danielson MD, Hoenig JM, Davis Jack SP, Brody DJ, Gyawali S, Maenner MM, Warner M, Holland KM, Perou R, Crosby AE, Blumberg SJ, Avenevoli S, Kaminski JW, Ghandour RM. Surveillance of Children's mental health—United States, 2013—2019. MMWR. 2022;71(Suppl-2):1–42.
2. Martini R, Hilt R, Marx L, et al. Best principles for integration of child psychiatry into the pediatric health home. 2012. This reference provides guidelines for best practices for integration of child and adolescent psychiatrists into pediatric primary care practices.
3. Cwik MF, O'Keefe VM, Haroz EE. Suicide in the pediatric population: screening, risk assessment and treatment. Int Rev Psychiatry. 2020;32(3):254–64. https://doi.org/10.1080/0954026 1.2019.1693351.
4. Hawes MT, Szenczy AK, Klein DN, Hajcak G, Nelson BD. Increases in depression and anxiety symptoms in adolescents and young adults during the COVID-19 pandemic. Psychol Med. 2021;13:1–9. https://doi.org/10.1017/S0033291720005358.
5. Mayne SL, Hannan C, Davis M, Young JF, Kelly MK, Powell M, Dalembert G, McPeak KE, Jenssen BP, Fiks AG. COVID-19 and adolescent depression and suicide risk screening outcomes. Pediatrics. 2021;148(3):e2021051507. https://doi.org/10.1542/peds.2021-051507.
6. Jones EAK, Mitra AK, Bhuiyan AR. Impact of COVID-19 on mental health in adolescents: a systematic review. Int J Environ Res Public Health. 2021;18(5):2470. https://doi.org/10.3390/ijerph18052470.
7. Racine N, McArthur BA, Cooke JE, Eirich R, Zhu J, Madigan S. Global prevalence of depressive and anxiety symptoms in children and adolescents during COVID-19: a meta-analysis. JAMA Pediatr. 2021;175(11):1142–50. https://doi.org/10.1001/jamapediatrics.2021.2482.

8. Hoffnung G, Feigenbaum E, Schechter A, Guttman D, Zemon V, Schechter I. Children and telehealth in mental healthcare: what we have learned from COVID-19 and 40,000+ sessions. Psychiatr Res Clin Pract. 2021;27 https://doi.org/10.1176/appi.prcp.20200035.
9. Molfenter T, Heitkamp T, Murphy AA, Tapscott S, Behlman S, Cody OJ. Use of telehealth in mental health (MH) services during and after COVID-19. Community Ment Health J. 2021;57(7):1244–51. https://doi.org/10.1007/s10597-021-00861-2.
10. Frank HE, Grumbach NM, Conrad SM, Wheeler J, Wolff J. Mental health services in primary care: evidence for the feasibility of telehealth during the COVID-19 pandemic. J Affect Disord Rep. 2021;5:100146. https://doi.org/10.1016/j.jadr.2021.100146.
11. Zuckerbrot RA, Cheung A, Jensen PS, Stein REK, Laraque D, GLAD-PC Steering Group. Guidelines for adolescent depression in primary care (GLAD-PC): part I. Practice preparation, identification, assessment, and initial management. Pediatrics. 2018;141(3):e20174081.
12. Gibbons RD, Brown CH, Hur K, Marcus SM, Bhaumik DK, Erkens JA, Herings RM, Mann JJ. Early evidence on the effects of regulators' suicidality warnings on SSRI prescriptions and suicide in children and adolescents. Am J Psychiatry. 2007;164(9):1356–63. https://doi.org/10.1176/appi.ajp.2007.07030454.
13. American Psychiatric Association. Diagnostic and statistical manual of mental disorders. 5th ed. Arlington, VA: American Psychiatric Association; 2013.
14. Maslow GR, Dunlap K, Chung RJ. Depression and suicide in children and adolescents. Pediatr Rev. 2015;36(7):299–310.
15. March JS, Silva S, Petrycki S, Curry J, Wells K, Fairbank J, Burns B, Domino M, McNulty S, Vitiello B, Severe J. The treatment for adolescents with depression study (TADS): long-term effectiveness and safety outcomes. Arch Gen Psychiatry. 2007;64(10):1132–43.
16. Shain B, Committee on Adolescence, Braverman PK, Adelman WP, Alderman EM, Breuner CC, Levine DA, Marcell AV, O'Brien RF. Suicide and suicide attempts in adolescents. Pediatrics. 2016;138(1):e20161420.
17. Hoge E, Bickham D, Cantor J. Digital media, anxiety, and depression in children. Pediatrics. 2017;140(Suppl 2):S76–80. https://doi.org/10.1542/peds.2016-1758G.
18. Bushnell GA, Compton SN, Dusetzina SB, et al. Treating pediatric anxiety: initial use of SSRIs and other antianxiety prescription medications. J Clin Psychiatry. 2018;79(1):16m11415. https://doi.org/10.4088/JCP.16m11415.
19. Bagnell AL. Anxiety and separation disorders. Pediatr Rev. 2011;32(10):440–6.
20. Siegel RS, Dickstein DP. Anxiety in adolescents: update on its diagnosis and treatment for primary care providers. Adolesc Health Med Ther. 2011;3:1–16. https://doi.org/10.2147/AHMT.S7597.
21. Kertz S, Bigda-Peyton J, Bjorgvinsson T. Validity of the generalized anxiety disorder-7 scale in an acute psychiatric sample. Clin Psychol Psychother. 2013;20:456–64.
22. Stahl SM. Stahl's essential psychopharmacology: prescriber's guide, children and adolescents. 1st ed. Cambridge: University Printing House; 2019.
23. Franchini L, Serretti A, Gasperini M, Smeraldi E. Familial concordance of fluvoxamine response as a tool for differentiating mood disorder pedigrees. J Psychiatr Res. 1998;32(5):255–9.
24. Southammakosane C, Schmitz K. Pediatric psychopharmacology for treatment of ADHD, depression, and anxiety. Pediatrics. 2015;136(2):351–9. https://doi.org/10.1542/peds.2014-1581.
25. Marken PA, Munro JS. Selecting a selective serotonin reuptake inhibitor: clinically important distinguishing features. Prim Care Companion J Clin Psychiatry. 2000;2(6):205–10. https://doi.org/10.4088/pcc.v02n0602.
26. Kweon K, Kim HW. Effectiveness and safety of bupropion in children and adolescents with depressive disorders: a retrospective chart review. Clin Psychopharmacol Neurosci. 2019;17(4):537–41. https://doi.org/10.9758/cpn.2019.17.4.537.
27. Greene JP, Dawson R. School-based health Center model within the military health system: the role of the adolescent medicine physician. Mil Med. 2016;181(9):1046–9.

28. Sasangohar F, Bradshaw MR, Carlson MM, et al. Adapting an outpatient psychiatric clinic to telehealth during the COVID-19 pandemic: a practice perspective. J Med Internet Res. 2020;22(10):e22523. https://doi.org/10.2196/22523.
29. Keks N, Hope J, Keogh S. Switching and stopping antidepressants. Aust Prescr. 2016;39(3):76–83.
30. Jha MK, Rush AJ, Trivedi MH. When discontinuing SSRI antidepressants is a challenge: management tips. Am J Psychiatry. 2018;175(12):1176–84.
31. Volpi-Abadie J, Kaye AM, Kaye AD. Serotonin syndrome. Ochsner J. 2013;13(4):533–40.

Chapter 11
Telemedicine for the Provision of Gender-Affirming Care for Trans Youth

Carolina Silva, Smita Mukherjee, and Brenden E. Hursh

Illustrative Case Examples

Case 1

Lily (she/her) is 12 years old and was assigned male at birth. She identifies as a girl and has used her affirmed name and pronouns since the age of 8 years. Over the last few months, she has noticed signs of pubertal development, and these changes are causing her significant distress. Lily's parents would like to have more information about puberty blockers and medical transition. They had a visit with their family doctor, who has known Lily for years and is willing to support her care. This local provider does not have any previous experience with gender-related care, but they offered to make a referral to a specialized center. Lily and her parents live in a rural community, and the closest pediatric gender clinic is a 7-hour drive away. This clinic has a waitlist of around 9 months, so she would be due for her appointment in the winter. The family is not sure that they will be able to attend then, because of the unfavorable road conditions during those months

Case 2

Jace (he/him) is a 17-year-old transmasculine person. He struggles with depression and anxiety. He has been receiving gender-affirming hormone therapy for almost 2 years and is followed by a multidisciplinary team in a tertiary care hospital. Jace is going through a difficult time in terms of his mental health. He has expressed his desire to continue his current hormone treatment, but he has missed a couple of clinic visits lately. Unfortunately, Jace had an unpleasant experience at the hospital laboratory last year while interacting with a staff member who had not received training in gender diversity, and he has not attended a hospital visit since then. His mom recently reached out to Jace's gender clinic, hoping to discuss alternative options for Jace to connect with his endocrinologist and multidisciplinary team

C. Silva · B. E. Hursh (✉)
Division of Endocrinology, BC Children's Hospital, Vancouver, BC, Canada

Department of Pediatrics, University of British Columbia, Vancouver, Canada
e-mail: carolina.silva@cw.bc.ca; brenden.hursh@cw.bc.ca

S. Mukherjee
Department of Urologic Sciences, University of British Columbia, Vancouver, BC, Canada

Gender Surgery Program, Vancouver Coastal Health, Vancouver, BC, Canada
e-mail: smita.mukherjee@ubc.ca

© The Author(s), under exclusive license to Springer Nature Switzerland AG 2024
Y. N. Evans et al. (eds.), *Telemedicine for Adolescent and Young Adult Health Care*, https://doi.org/10.1007/978-3-031-55760-6_11

Key Points

Telemedicine for Gender-Affirming Care—Key Points
- Gender-affirming care has been associated with significant benefits for trans youth; however, there are several challenges to accessing this care
- Telemedicine could help overcome many of the barriers to care that trans youth face
- Telemedicine can facilitate collaborative multidisciplinary, multicenter care and capacity building for local healthcare providers
- Delivery of gender-affirming care via telemedicine significantly increased during the COVID-19 pandemic
- Trans youth and families report positive experiences and are asking for inclusion of telemedicine in their future care
- Ongoing evaluation of experiences and outcomes of telemedicine-delivered gender care is needed

---

Transgender Identities: Definition and Prevalence

"Transgender" (or "trans") is an umbrella definition to describe individuals who have gender identities that are not aligned with their sex recorded at birth [1]. People whose gender identities fall between, beyond, or outside the conventional male or female normative roles may choose expressions such as "non-binary," "gender-diverse," and "genderqueer," among others [2–4]. Within some Indigenous communities, the term "Two-Spirit" is used to reflect their complex notion of gender roles and history of gender diversity [5]. We use "trans youth" to encompass adolescents and young adults with a broad spectrum of gender identities, understanding that these may be subject to change over time. The estimated proportion of transgender identities has been reported to range between 0.5% and 3% [6, 7]. However, this may be higher at younger ages, as gender incongruence in prepubertal children does not always persist later in life [8]. There also appears to be a trend toward higher percentages seen in recent years, with a recent study showing that up to 9% of adolescents report gender-diverse identities [9].

Gender dysphoria is defined as the distress caused by the discrepancy between a person's gender identity and their sex assigned at birth, which impacts social, occupational, or other important areas of functioning [10, 11]. Only some transgender and gender-nonconforming people experience gender dysphoria at some point in their lives, and the proportion of children and adolescents who do so is not well known [10].

Gender-Affirming Care for Trans Youth: An Overview

Trans youth deserve gender-affirming care options and access to health care that aligns with their needs. The World Professional Association for Transgender Health and the Endocrine Society, among other expert groups, have published consensus guidelines on the provision of such care [10, 12]. It is important to consider that these are general recommendations, as one of the main principles of gender-affirming care is that it needs to be tailored to each youth's individual needs and goals. In addition, gender affirmation involves numerous aspects, such as supporting trans youth to present socially in their affirmed gender role, and it may (or may not) include providing medical or surgical interventions. There is broad agreement that the care of trans youth requires a multidisciplinary approach. This usually involves mental health professionals, endocrinologists, pediatricians or adolescent medicine specialists, family physicians and nurse practitioners, nurses, social workers, surgeons, gynecologists, fertility specialists, and other members of the healthcare team, depending on each person's needs [10, 12, 13].

Medical treatment for trans youth includes pubertal suppression and hormone therapy. Experiencing physical changes that are not aligned with a person's gender identity can be seriously distressing. Gonadotropin-releasing hormone (GnRH) analogs, commonly known as "puberty blockers," prevent the development or progression of such undesired secondary sexual characteristics. The main intention of this therapy is to provide trans youth more time to explore their gender identity and define their goals regarding physical transition without experiencing nonreversible body changes [10, 12, 14]. GnRH analogs are administered via intramuscular or subcutaneous injections or as a subcutaneous implant. Treatment can be initiated soon after the onset of puberty, when a youth reaches Tanner stage 2 [10, 12]. This is a reversible intervention, and stopping therapy, if appropriate, will lead to the resumption of endogenous puberty. While there is paucity of long-term outcome studies in trans youth, available information continues to support the safety and efficacy of GnRH analogs [10, 12, 15, 16]. For individuals who pursue gender-affirming care after their pubertal development is complete, GnRH analogs can be used as an option to stop menses or to prevent facial hair growth, but this treatment would not revert most physical changes that have already occurred.

Hormone therapy induces the development of secondary sex characteristics that are aligned with a person's gender identity. Clinical practice guidelines recommend consideration of hormone therapy once a youth has the capacity to provide informed consent [10, 12]. While current guidelines support the initiation of hormone treatment at age 16, these also acknowledge some risks associated with postponing therapy until then, and that treatment may be considered at younger ages in certain situations [10, 12]. Prolonged pubertal suppression may have detrimental effects on bone health, and there are also concerns about psychosocial consequences to trans youth, as most cisgender peers will have gone through puberty by this age. Thus, in many centers, hormone therapy is initiated at earlier ages [14, 17]. Dosing, choice of different formulations, and routes of administration vary widely. Estrogen can be delivered orally, transdermally, or (less commonly) by injection, and common methods of administration of testosterone include injections (intramuscular or subcutaneous), topical gel and patches. In general, hormone therapy for trans youth is started at relatively low doses and is gradually increased, mimicking the physiologic progression of puberty. This can be combined with GnRH agonists or other treatments, such as anti-androgen medications, to reduce the expression of masculinizing physical features in those assigned male at birth. For those assigned female at birth, various alternatives for menstrual suppression are available, such as oral combined contraceptives, progesterone-only pills, medroxyprogesterone injections, and progesterone-containing intrauterine or implantable devices [10, 12, 18].

Gender-affirming surgeries include procedures to change primary and/or secondary sex characteristics (breasts/chest, external and/or internal genitalia, facial features, body contouring), which aim to alleviate gender dysphoria, by assisting trans people with achieving comfort with their body and identity [10]. For those assigned male at birth, gender-affirming surgeries include breast augmentation, vaginoplasty, vulvoplasty, penectomy, orchiectomy, and feminizing facial surgeries. People assigned female at birth may choose to undergo chest reconstruction surgery, oophorectomy, hysterectomy, phalloplasty, or metoidioplasty. In most countries, gender-affirming surgery is typically limited to older youth and adults, but adolescents may have access to some of these procedures on a case-by-case basis [10, 12, 19].

Trans youth and their families should also have access to appropriate psychosocial supports [20]. Medical and surgical treatments are provided to trans youth who are diagnosed with gender dysphoria or gender incongruence by a trained, trans-competent professional [10, 12]. It is essential to ensure that mental health care is not only available for such initial comprehensive assessment or care planning, but also throughout their journey. Approaches that do not pathologize gender diversity and that do promote free exploration and self-definition have been associated with significantly better outcomes [20, 21]. The gender-affirmative model defines gender health as the opportunity to live in the gender that feels most real or comfortable and to express that without criticism or rejection [22].

Medical visits for gender-affirming care for youth usually involve an endocrinologist, adolescent medicine specialist, or another trans-competent healthcare provider. During initial visits, providers obtain information about the youth's medical history, discuss goals in terms of physical body changes, and review risks and benefits from therapy with the youth and family, so they can make an informed decision. As a part of these conversations, fertility preservation should be discussed before initiating puberty blockers and hormone therapy [10, 12, 23]. A physical exam for evaluation of pubertal status may be performed before initiation of treatment, as GnRH analogs are only indicated after the onset of puberty; however, a thorough medical history and laboratory measured hormone levels could also indicate pubertal onset [10, 12]. Regular follow-up visits are intended to review the progress with current medical therapy, side effects, and future goals. On many occasions, laboratory investigations, including gonadotropin and sex steroid levels, in addition to the trans youth's report, can provide accurate information about the suppression of the gonadal axis and/or adequacy of hormone therapy, without the need for a physical examination. This is particularly relevant given that chest and genital exams can be quite distressing for this population.

During gender-care visits, several other aspects of general adolescent health (social determinants of health, physical activity and eating habits, emotional well-being, substance use, reproductive health and sexually transmitted infection prevention, etc.) are also addressed. Allied healthcare team members are usually involved in gender-related visits, particularly at specialized centers, aiming to provide comprehensive care to trans youth and families. When necessary, youth and caregivers learn how to self-administer medications (including subcutaneous or intramuscular injections). Gender visits may also be an opportunity to discuss other aspects, such as legal name or gender marker changes, resources for social transition, and school support.

Vulnerability, Minority Stress, and Mental Health of Trans Youth

Unfortunately, stigma and prejudice around gender diversity are still seen in many societies. Despite increasing social visibility and legal recognition over the past years, a significant proportion of trans youth experience discrimination because of their gender identity at some point during their lives [24–27]. Many of them face such issues at their own homes or school, which may explain the higher rates of homelessness and lower levels of education seen in this population [25, 26]. Difficulties obtaining employment are further accentuated by workplace discrimination, as well as laws and policies that deny gender recognition [26–28]. For instance, in many countries, trans people do not have access to documentation that is congruent with their gender identity [26, 29].

Trans youth are clearly a vulnerable population. This group is more likely to face bullying and harassment than their cisgender peers [30–32]. Some studies have shown that trans youth have higher rates of involvement in high-risk behaviors such as substance abuse and less protective factors than their cisgender counterparts [7, 33]. Physical violence and sexual harassment are commonly reported by trans youth [24, 32, 34]. The prevalence of HIV infection is still unfairly high among transgender individuals, particularly trans women [35, 36].

Further, trans youth also experience notable mental health disparities. A significant proportion of this group struggles with anxiety and/or depression [24, 37–39]. Self-injury and suicidality are serious concerns, with substantially higher rates occurring in trans youth compared to their cisgender peers [24, 38–40]. Eating disorders are also disproportionately seen in this population [41]. There is no evidence that gender identity inherently places trans youth at risk for mental health problems. It appears that this increased risk is associated with several adverse external factors, in addition to gender dysphoria. Such elements, related to gender minority stress, include discrimination, rejection, non-affirmation, internalized transphobia, and non-disclosure [20, 42–44]. On the other hand, affirming relationships with parents and family and social supports and safety at school have been highlighted as resilience-promoting factors for trans youth [7, 45].

Moreover, there continue to be significant challenges for trans youth to access medical care [46–49]. Many of these difficulties arise from discrimination and systemic barriers. Several reports have revealed trans people's negative experiences and concerns about the healthcare system [47–49]. A study among trans youth in Canada showed that they are not receiving the medical attention that they feel they need [24]. Likewise, in a survey conducted in the United States, one in every four trans individuals stated that they avoid seeking care due to fear of being mistreated [26]. Trans youth frequently worry about having their gender identity mocked or dismissed by the healthcare team, or their confidentiality being breached by providers disclosing their gender identity to other staff members [50–52]. Additionally, this group has raised concerns about being asked irrelevant questions or being exposed to unnecessary examinations during gender-unrelated medical visits [52, 53].

Importance of Gender-Affirming Care

Being able to explore gender identity and expression both freely and with adequate support can lead to substantial improvement in overall quality of life and well-being. Studies have shown that trans youth who are supported in their gender identity and have transitioned socially have notably better psychosocial outcomes [54]. Being able to use their chosen name is associated with reduced rates of depression, anxiety, and even suicidal ideation [55]. Considering this, receiving care which follows a gender-affirmative care model and which validates gender identity, experience, emotions and goals can have a profound impact.

Over the past years, there has been increasing evidence regarding the beneficial effects of gender-affirming medical treatment. In general, trans youth perceive the care provided at specialty gender clinics as helpful [56]. Receiving puberty blockers or hormone therapy can lead to improved mental health outcomes soon after these treatments are started [57, 58]. Various studies have demonstrated that, once they start treatment with GnRH analogs, trans youth have fewer behavioral and emotional problems and that their psychological functioning is equivalent or better to their cisgender peers [59–61]. In addition, trans youth receiving pubertal suppression appear to have a lower risk of suicidal ideation compared to those who desire such treatment but are not receiving it [62]. Similarly, receiving hormone therapy can lead to lower rates of depression and suicidality among trans youth [63, 64]. On the other side, barriers to accessing medical transition may lead to increased stress and worsening mental health outcomes in this population [56, 65]. These are powerful findings, which highlight the importance of ensuring access to gender-affirming care.

As a final note regarding provision of gender-affirming care to trans children and youth: this care is unique in that the timing of interventions intersects directly with the timing of puberty to determine physical outcomes. In addition to the powerful psychological and social impacts for a youth of pausing pubertal changes that do not align with their gender identity, GnRH agonists can also improve physical outcomes when initiated at earlier stages of puberty [19, 66]. For instance, transfeminine youth do not experience deepening of their voice or development of a laryngeal prominence, male bone configuration, or noticeable androgen-dependent hair growth, if treatment is started soon after puberty onset. Similarly, transmasculine youth treated early with puberty blockers may have less significant breast development, reducing the need for chest masculinizing surgeries or improving surgical outcomes for those who undergo such procedures [15, 67].

Challenges to the Provision of Gender-Affirming Care

The number of trans youth being referred to gender clinics in North America and Europe has experienced a steep rise over the past decade, and it continues to show an upward trend [68–70]. Nevertheless, inequities persist, and trans youth still face many barriers to accessing care.

One of the most important difficulties is the paucity of trans-competent healthcare providers [71–73]. Currently, the conventional medical curricula does not generally include adequate instruction in transgender health [74, 75]. Thus, many physicians and members of the healthcare team complete their general or specialty training without achieving basic competence in providing care to trans individuals. There is a shortage of medical and mental health professionals with adequate knowledge and skills to provide gender-affirming care [76]. To date, most gender clinics have lengthy waitlists, and many trans youth need to wait months or even more than a year for their first clinic visit [77]. This can be quite disappointing and stressful, particularly while they are awaiting time-sensitive interventions such as initiation of puberty blockers.

Additionally, gender-affirming care is mostly delivered in specialized clinics located in large urban centers [78, 79]. Attending gender clinic visits in-person can be quite burdensome to some families, as they need to consider the time and expenses associated with traveling to the clinic, parking, taking time off work or school and arranging for childcare, and organizing their schedules around appointment times that are not usually very flexible. Indeed, almost one-third of trans youth across Canada mentioned transportation as a barrier to receiving adequate gender-affirming care [24]. In a recent survey, a significant proportion of trans youth and caregivers mentioned that they would miss a half or full day of work or school, and they would need to spend considerable amounts of money to attend an in-person gender-related visit [80]. It is not surprising that trans youth living in rural and remote areas are unfairly underrepresented in pediatric gender clinics [81, 82].

Furthermore, many trans youth and their families also face financial hardships related to the cost of healthcare visits and treatments. Gender-affirming care is not explicitly addressed in legislation in many countries and states, leading to legal and insurance-associated barriers to care [26, 83]. Even in countries with universal healthcare and inclusive policies, the cost of medications, particularly puberty blockers, can be prohibitive. Many localities have very limited free or accessible options for psychological support, counseling, and similar resources, which are essential components of multidisciplinary gender-affirming care. Likewise, fertility preservation is rarely covered by government or private healthcare insurers. Thus, trans youth from under-resourced households are often unable to access these important aspects of care. Housing instability or mental health challenges, which affect a substantial proportion of trans youth, impose an additional layer of complexity to this difficult scenario [72].

Parental support may also significantly impact a trans youth's likelihood of receiving gender-affirming care. Needing to "come out" to parents and family members has been identified by this group as a barrier to accessing care [56]. In many countries, the current legislation requires parental consent for the provision of gender-related care, and even if this is not formally needed to deliver care, it might not be easy for a trans youth to navigate the medical system on their own. Some youth may completely depend on their family to attend a clinic visit because they live far away and/or they are too young to travel on their own. This certainly exacerbates the inequities between trans youth with and without family and financial support.

The COVID-19 pandemic added further obstacles to accessing gender-affirming care. With the onset of this pandemic, a significant number of in-person appointments deemed "non-urgent" were cancelled or postponed, and many patients avoided attending healthcare settings due to fear of contracting COVID-19. Therefore, it became even harder for trans individuals to access medical care and gender-affirming surgeries. During this time, concerns about mental distress grew considerably, and access to mental health support was reduced, exacerbating previous disparities for this population [84]. Moreover, the economic impact of the pandemic worsened the financial struggles of already marginalized groups, and those who lost their jobs or saw their income reduced during this time likely faced additional difficulties accessing care.

Finally, even when access is possible, trans youth may not be willing or able to engage with the medical system, due to real or perceived discrimination [7, 47, 72]. While gender clinics intend to be inclusive spaces, healthcare environments are not always perceived as safe by the trans population [71]. Trans youth have reported mistreatment and unpleasant experiences in waiting rooms, and many are afraid of being seen receiving gender-related care because of stigma associated with being gender diverse [56, 78]. Most hospitals still have gender-segregated spaces and do not have widespread availability of gender-neutral washrooms. In addition, many healthcare settings lack adequate staff training on gender diversity, and youth have highlighted that nonmedical staff and healthcare providers, particularly in hospital areas outside the gender clinic, use incorrect names and pronouns with them [56, 71, 85]. Medical records and even identification wristbands often display a name that the youth no longer identifies with, which can cause significant distress [53]. Although there is growing adaptation of inclusive electronic medical records, many hospital forms contain binary language or collect information on biological sex instead of gender, and similarly, growth charts and laboratory reports use sex-based references, all of which can lead to misunderstandings and uncomfortable situations for trans youth. Understandably, these negative experiences exacerbate vulnerability and lead to mistrust of the medical system, pushing trans youth further away.

Telemedicine for the Provision of Gender-Affirming Care: Potential Benefits

Benefits of Telemedicine for Gender-Affirming Care
- Increased access to experienced providers and high-quality care
- Reduced cost and burden associated with attending medical visits (transportation, time off work or school)
- Easier delivery of collaborative, multidisciplinary care
- Capacity building for local providers
- Improved safety of visits for trans youth
- Decreased likelihood of discrimination in healthcare settings
- Positive experience for youth and family

Telemedicine has the potential to overcome many of the challenges that trans youth face to receiving appropriate care. Indeed, several studies have shown that telemedicine visits are feasible and can increase access to gender-affirming care [86–89]. During the COVID-19 pandemic, telemedicine enabled the provision of gender-affirming care for this population. Not only has this model ensured continuity of patient care, but also, a considerable number of new patients were seen across different gender clinics via telemedicine [86, 89]. Additionally, during this time, access to telehealth-delivered gender-affirming care showed a positive effect on mental health outcomes of trans people [90].

One of the most important benefits of telemedicine visits is reducing barriers resulting from the limited number of multidisciplinary gender clinics and their placement in larger urban centers. With this modality, trans youth can receive care regardless of their geographic location. Furthermore, telemedicine provides an easier, less time-consuming, and less expensive option for the delivery of care, which is of key importance given the access disparities seen in this group. This is also relevant considering that gender-affirming care usually involves multidisciplinary care. Coordinating multiple visits can be quite burdensome, particularly if different specialists do not practice in the same location, and this would become simpler if trans youth and their family did not need to travel to a healthcare facility for each appointment [78, 86]. Similarly, education sessions and interactions with other team members (e.g., social worker or nurse) via telemedicine could be arranged separately from clinician visits, on the same or a different day, providing more flexibility and allowing for efficient use of resources. When appropriate, telemedicine may also facilitate participation of family members and caregivers in these visits, even if they are in different locations, which can potentially enhance their engagement with the youth's medical care and support. Another intriguing aspect of telemedicine care is that trans youth may attend visits on their own, without needing to rely on a parent for transportation. As expected, trans youth with lower perceived parental support seem to be particularly interested in being able to receive gender-affirming care via telemedicine [91].

Moreover, there are many local healthcare providers (family physicians, nurse practitioners, pediatricians) who follow trans youth and who may already have a non-gender-related relationship with them; these providers may be very willing to contribute with certain aspects of their care, but lack the expertise or a multidisciplinary team needed to provide comprehensive gender-affirming care. Telemedicine can facilitate collaboration between local providers and distant specialists in larger centers [91, 92]. This model of care could allow for support in the co-management of these youth, with specialists sharing knowledge and experience and providing guidance in more complex situations [92]. This would not only be an excellent example of youth- and family-centered care, but may also reduce the burden on specialized multidisciplinary gender clinics, most of which are finding it difficult to increase their capacity to see new patients to keep up with increasing referrals. At the same time, this collaborative model would give local healthcare providers the opportunity to gain skills and knowledge in gender-affirming care and to create networks with specialty clinics. Such capacity building may lead to general practitioners being able to provide care to a larger group of trans people and, ultimately, contribute to the sustainability of "communities of care" within the local health system. Additionally, telemedicine has the potential to improve access to allied healthcare team members, such as social workers, counsellors, etc., who could work together with primary care providers in a true multidisciplinary, collaborative fashion.

Another potential benefit of telemedicine for gender-affirming care is that it can provide a safe environment. Trans youth who participated in telemedicine gender-related visits reported these to be as safe or safer than in-person care [80, 93]. Moreover, they described telemedicine visits as more comfortable, and they expressed feeling less anxious during these visits. The reasons for these findings may be multiple. Telemedicine may reduce the stress associated with attending a healthcare setting that might be perceived as non-inclusive. In certain situations, for example, in smaller communities, it can be quite challenging to protect a person's anonymity while receiving gender-affirming care. Telemedicine may be perceived as safer by trans youth who fear being "outed" by attending a gender clinic. The opportunity of joining visits alone (compared to attending in-person visits with a parent or a caregiver) could also be beneficial in regard to their safety. By allowing trans youth to receive care from their home or a comfortable location, telemedicine could be helpful to those youth who lack family support and for whom traveling to a healthcare center to receive gender-affirming care might be challenging. Considering the vulnerability of this population, the opportunity of delivering care in a way that is perceived as safe cannot be overlooked.

Telemedicine for the Delivery of Gender-Affirming Care: Opportunities

Internet and social media are widely used by trans youth to share experiences, learn about each others' journeys, and find support from peers and allies. As the health system can be quite difficult to navigate, trans youth often choose to look for resources and learn about medical treatments and surgeries online, understanding (or not) that some of this information may not be entirely accurate [94–96]. In this context, being able to connect with knowledgeable, trans-competent providers online and to obtain reliable information could be extremely valuable for this group [53].

Telemedicine can be useful for the provision of many different aspects of care for trans youth. Given the nature of gender-affirming care, our experience is that physical exams play a relatively minor role in a health care visit, while the opportunity to engage with trans youth and their family is of utmost importance. General aspects of adolescent health can certainly be discussed over telemedicine. Mental health assessments are a very good example of visits that can be successfully delivered via telemedicine [97, 98]. This may also be the case for many other specialist medical visits, with physical exam components arranged with local providers, when needed. Particularly regarding medical gender-affirming therapy, initiating puberty blockers may require someone competent in assessing how far along someone is in puberty; however, indications for hormone treatment are often established by youth and family report, and contraindications are usually identified by medical history or investigations [10, 12, 78, 99]. This therapy may be safely prescribed after a telemedicine assessment with a specialist, provided that a local health practitioner is able to obtain laboratory testing, perform a physical exam and obtain anthropometric measurements and vital signs. Likewise, puberty blockers and hormone therapy can be adequately monitored through history and laboratory testing in most cases, as long as the youth also has ongoing in-person visits arranged locally, as required, for general health checkups. For some surgical interventions, the initial evaluation, conversations about different approaches, risks and benefits, and the consent process may be successfully performed via telemedicine. Similarly, part or all post-procedure follow-up could be by telemedicine, if there is a local practitioner that can provide general care. This would vastly decrease the need for in-person specialist visits, with their associated costs and barriers [78].

Telemedicine may also be an option to connect with trans youth who are awaiting a gender-affirming care visit. A visit with trans-competent providers (nurses and social workers, among others) via telemedicine can be used to guide the youth and family who are trying to navigate the medical system and to facilitate the provision of resources for social transition, such as information for school or applying for legal name and gender marker change [100]. By helping trans youth and their families feel reassured, this may mitigate the negative effects of prolonged delays until their first medical visit [77]. Such telemedicine visits can also provide important information for triaging, based on the knowledge of the youth, their context, and available supports.

Importantly, trans youth seem to be interested in having telemedicine-delivered gender care. A study in the United States evaluating trans youth's preferences and values toward telemedicine showed highly encouraging responses [91]. Similarly, studies that assessed the experiences of trans youth and their families with telemedicine for gender care during the COVID-19 pandemic revealed very good usability of these visits and overall positive perceptions with high rates of satisfaction [80, 86, 93, 99]. Many trans youth and their caregivers feel that telemedicine visits are equivalent to, or better than in-person visits for gender-affirming care [80, 99]. Among other findings, trans youth reported that it is easy to communicate with their doctor using telemedicine and that they can express themselves effectively [80]. It was also highlighted that some youth may find it easier to engage in open conversations with their providers virtually, compared to face-to-face interactions [86].

Many trans youth are hopeful to have telemedicine as a part of their future care [80, 99]. It appears that a combination of telemedicine and in-person visits is the most desired model of care moving forward [80]. Preferences and attitudes toward telemedicine may vary depending on the specific purpose of the visit, and it is essential to consider this to provide care that is individualized to each person's context and needs. For instance, in-person encounters may still be preferred over telemedicine for first-time medical visits, as well as for surgical planning or teaching how to self-administer injections [91, 93]. Ongoing evaluation of the experience and health outcomes of youth who continue to receive gender-affirming care via telemedicine is needed.

Telemedicine Visits for Gender-Affirming Care: Challenges

Despite all the advantageous aspects of telemedicine-delivered gender-affirming care, some pitfalls need to be considered. First, access to a computer with reliable Internet connection or a smart device with data are required. In addition, while many platforms used for telemedicine are user-friendly, families need to have a basic level of technological expertise to be able to participate in such visits. These factors can be a barrier for socially or financially under-resourced trans youth, or for those living in remote communities. Furthermore, the lack of safe and private spaces to have a telemedicine visit is an important concern [78]. This is particularly relevant in gender-related visits, where sensitive topics are discussed. Trans youth should have the opportunity to disclose in confidence mental health concerns, bullying, and intimate partner violence and discuss other topics such as sexual and reproductive health or substance use; not having an ensured safe space for the visit further perpetuates disparities in an already vulnerable group.

One aspect of telemedicine that may need special attention in these youth is possible dysphoria related to seeing their image on the screen. In our practice, it is not uncommon that trans youth turn their cameras off or stay distant from the computer during telemedicine visits. Studies assessing trans youths' experiences have also pointed this out as a concern [90]. In addition, while it is likely that younger generations have different and evolving views about connecting virtually, telemedicine visits may still lead to difficulties in developing youth-provider rapport. Both trans youth and their families have described that it is harder to establish a relationship with their doctor over telemedicine visits [80, 86]. It appears that those who never met with their team in person find it harder to build bonds and trust [80].

Furthermore, although many gender-related visits can be conducted via telemedicine, this model may not entirely replace in-person visits. As mentioned, confirmation of pubertal status is required to initiate GnRH analogs, and in some situations, this may be best facilitated by physical exam. Even when hormone or blocker therapy is monitored by history and laboratory investigations, evaluation of general health may require an in-person physical exam, e.g., to obtain height, weight, and blood pressure measurements. Trans youth who receive care via telemedicine will still need to attend healthcare settings for laboratory testing, as well as surgical procedures and immediate post-procedure follow-up. Additionally, receiving teaching on how to administer subcutaneous or intramuscular injections may be easier if this is provided in person, as educators may have more hands-on resources to teach, and some families might feel more reassured with in-person supervision and guidance while they are giving their first injections.

Important Considerations and Tips for Successful Delivery of Telemedicine Gender-Related Care

Practical Tips for Successful Telemedicine Visits for Gender Care
Ensure a welcoming environment in preparation and, during the visit, use of correct pronouns and name
Allow youth to disable self-view if it is distressing for them to see their own image on screen
Identify all attendees in the visit and their pronouns. Ask explicitly about participants off-camera
Confirm with trans youth the safety of their environment. If needed, use nonverbal communication and/or chat features
Include family members as appropriate but also allow for one-on-one time
Facilitate space for a private, confidential discussion with trans youth
Create a plan for investigations and physical exams to be performed locally, if required

There are several options to facilitate the delivery of gender care via telemedicine. To begin with, families must receive clear instructions in preparation for their visits, and when needed, technical support should be available. Phone visits could be an alternative to address issues regarding Internet connection, smartphone or computer ownership, and technological literacy. Another alternative to address these challenges is to facilitate telemedicine visits at schools, libraries, or local healthcare centers.

Establishing an affirming and welcoming environment is crucial for successful delivery of gender-related care [51]. To achieve this, clinic staff should have adequate cultural competency training when working with trans people. Asking and documenting chosen names and pronouns are paramount, as well as providing inclusive communications to youth and families [85, 101]. Protocols around laboratory requisitions and other medical forms with legal names should be reviewed, to ensure trans youth and families understand the limitations of the current healthcare system and so that these are not perceived as intentional forms of discrimination. While this certainly applies to in-person visits as well, it is possible that making mistakes of this kind might be harder to overcome when youth are not seen in person and do not have a relationship with clinic staff.

In general, telemedicine visits should include video technology (instead of audio only), as this can be helpful to generate empathy and trust and, ultimately, contribute to building a relationship with the trans youth and family [78, 102]. At the same time, it should be taken into consideration that, for some trans youth, seeing themselves on camera might cause significant distress [93]. Offering to disable the self-view feature, but still allowing youth to view the provider, can be a potential solution, and phone calls may be another alternative. Instructions for youth and families who are awaiting their first telemedicine visits should explicitly mention this possibility for those who do not feel comfortable with video technology. Although in-person meetings are certainly not required in all cases, alternating between in-person and telemedicine visits may contribute to strengthening connections, particularly early on in the youth-provider relationship [86]. Other possible strategies to build rapport with youth via telemedicine include starting conversations about shared interests such as hobbies, pets, artwork, or collectibles and, if appropriate, providing the opportunity to show these on camera [86].

To protect youth's safety and privacy, secure platforms should be used to deliver telemedicine, and providers should implement security measures and procedures to minimize potential privacy breaches [103, 104]. Importantly, youth should be asked if they are comfortable performing the visit in their current environment and if they are ready to start the visit. Ideally, this should be reviewed by clinic staff in preparation for their telemedicine visit and then discussed again with their provider at each encounter. Another good practice is to inquire about the presence of other people in the same room with the youth, who may be off camera or in adjacent rooms and could be listening. When there are concerns about privacy, enabling video technology may be helpful, as this allows for the use of nonverbal cues. In addition, most telemedicine platforms have a chat feature, which can provide a safe and private means of communication for youth who may be worried about other people listening to the conversation. Providers should also make sure that their environment is safe and respectful for the trans youth. Among other precautions, they should consider conducting the visit from a professional workspace, avoiding interruptions and background noise, and introducing other members of the healthcare team and learners if they are part of the visit. Confidentiality must be specifically discussed in this context. Participation of caregivers in gender-related visits is highly valuable, but at the same time, trans youth should not be denied the opportunity of having confidential conversations with their providers. During telemedicine visits, such conversations can be facilitated, for example, by asking the trans youth to move to another room for part of their appointment.

Finally, in terms of the lack of in-person examinations, there are several options. While initiation of puberty blockers requires confirmation of pubertal status, laboratory investigations can potentially be used instead of physical exams. Furthermore, vital signs such as height, weight, and blood pressure measurements may be obtained at local pharmacies or even at home, if the appropriate equipment is available [78]. In many cases, combining in-person and telemedicine visits can also be indicated. With this hybrid model, trans youth would have regular physical exams but, at the same time, would be able to connect with their team in an easier, more accessible way between in-person appointments. Trans youth exclusively seen by telemedicine at specialized gender clinics may benefit from being followed by family physicians, nurse practitioners, pediatricians, or other local providers who can see them in person closer to their homes and conduct such physical exams. Identifying ahead of time the need for blood tests and physical exams, and then partnering with local providers to facilitate these before the specialist telemedicine visit, has been found to be another effective solution [86].

Case Resolution

Case 1

Lily and her family will likely benefit from receiving gender-affirming care services via telemedicine. The distance to a multidisciplinary gender-affirming care center appears to be a significant challenge; however, Lily has a local practitioner who is willing to support her care. Connecting via telemedicine with the specialist team, while relying on her family physician for physical exams, growth monitoring, and even laboratory testing, can allow Lily to receive high-quality care that is also feasible and convenient for her family. This is crucial considering the significant distress that she is experiencing, as well as the potential benefits of timely initiation of puberty blockers. Moreover, her family doctor will have the chance to start building relationships with specialists in gender care and may gradually develop competency in the care of trans youth

Case 2

Telemedicine visits may also be a good alternative for Jace, who has not been able to attend in-person visits given his current mental health struggles. His negative experience being misgendered in the laboratory is possibly affecting his willingness to attend in-person care. Having the opportunity to have his visits via telemedicine from a safe and comfortable space may allow Jace to engage again with his healthcare team. It is clear that receiving gender-affirming care can positively impact mental health, and furthermore, additional psychosocial support can be also offered via telemedicine. In addition to ensuring ongoing care for Jace, it will be important to review hospital procedures and staff training with the goal of preventing further episodes of discrimination, whether intentional or unintentional, that could push trans youth away from the healthcare system

Conclusion

Telemedicine is a powerful tool, with the potential to overcome many barriers to accessing gender-affirming care for trans youth, such as distance to specialized centers, which are mainly located in large urban areas, and costs associated with attending a visit. Telemedicine-delivered gender care has been well-received, and trans youth and families who have been involved in such visits are generally satisfied. Telemedicine visits are perceived as safe, which is particularly relevant in this vulnerable group. By being able to connect with their providers from their home or a comfortable space, the fear of discrimination associated with attending healthcare centers may be alleviated. Furthermore, telemedicine provides the opportunity to build capacity of general practitioners and to create networks with specialized centers for the provision of collaborative and multidisciplinary care. One of the challenges with this model is the lack of physical examinations, which could be solved by partnering with local providers or combining telemedicine and in-person visits. The latter option may also help to strengthen relationships with trans youth, which may be difficult when using telemedicine alone. Successful delivery of gender care via telemedicine requires a welcoming environment and safe space for the youth. Offering to disable the self-viewing feature can be helpful for those who experience dysphoria from seeing themselves on the screen. It is also of key importance to continue to offer the opportunity to engage in private, confidential conversations with the youth during telemedicine visits.

Telemedicine presents many opportunities to expand and improve care of trans youth. As the model of telemedicine-delivered gender affirming health care continues to develop, it is essential to continue to gather information on the experiences of those involved and to assess their health care outcomes.

Acknowledgments We sincerely thank Dr. Daniel Metzger for his review of this manuscript and thoughtful feedback.

References

1. American Psychological Association. Guidelines for psychological practice with transgender and gender nonconforming people. Am Psychol. 2015;70:832–64. https://doi.org/10.1037/a0039906.
2. Thorne N, Yip AKT, Bouman WP, Marshall E, Arcelus J. The terminology of identities between, outside and beyond the gender binary—A systematic review. Int J Transgend. 2019;20:138–54. https://doi.org/10.1080/15532739.2019.1640654.
3. Scandurra C, Mezza F, Maldonato NM, Bottone M, Bochicchio V, Valerio P, et al. Health of nonbinary and genderqueer people: a systematic review. Front Psychol. 2019;10:1453. https://doi.org/10.3389/fpsyg.2019.01453.
4. Monro S. Non-binary and genderqueer: an overview of the field. Int J Transgend. 2019;20(2-3):126–31. https://doi.org/10.1080/15532739.2018.1538841.

5. Gender-affirming care for trans, two-spirit, and gender diverse patients in BC: A Primary Care Toolkit. TransCare BC 2021. Available from: http://www.phsa.ca/transcarebc/Documents/HealthProf/Primary-Care-Toolkit.pdf. Accessed 22 Apr 2022.
6. Sumia M, Lindberg N, Työläjärvi M, Kaltiala-Heino R. Current and recalled childhood gender identity in community youth in comparison to referred adolescents seeking sex reassignment. J Adolesc. 2017;56:34–9. https://doi.org/10.1016/j.adolescence.2017.01.006.
7. Eisenberg ME, Gower A, McMorris BJ, Nic Rider G, Shea G, Coleman E. Risk and protective factors in the lives of transgender/gender nonconforming adolescents. J Adolesc Health. 2017;61:521–6. https://doi.org/10.1016/j.jadohealth.2017.04.014.
8. Steensma TD, Biemond R, de Boer F, Cohen-Kettenis PT. Desisting and persisting gender dysphoria after childhood: a qualitative follow-up study. Clin Child Psychol Psychiatry. 2011;16(4):499–516. https://doi.org/10.1177/1359104510378303.
9. Kidd KM, Sequeira GM, Douglas C, Paglisotti T, Inwards-Breland DJ, Miller E, et al. Prevalence of gender-diverse youth in an urban school district. Pediatrics. 2021;147:e2020049823. https://doi.org/10.1542/peds.2020-049823.
10. Coleman E, Radix AE, Bouman WP, Brown GR, de Vries ALC, Deutsch MB, et al. Standards of care for the health of transgender and gender diverse people, Version 8. Int J Transgend Health. 2022;23(1):S1–S259. https://doi.org/10.1080/26895269.2022.2100644.
11. American Psychiatric Association. Diagnostic and statistical manual of mental disorders. 5th ed. Arlington: American Psychiatric Association; 2013.
12. Hembree WC, Cohen-Kettenis PT, Gooren L, Hannema SE, Meyer WJ, Murad MH, et al. Endocrine treatment of gender-dysphoric/gender-incongruent persons: an Endocrine Society Clinical Practice Guideline. Endocr Pract. 2017;23(12):1437. https://doi.org/10.4158/1934-2403-23.12.1437.
13. Chen D, Hidalgo MA, Leibowitz S, Chen D, Leininger J, Simons L, Finlayson C, et al. Multidisciplinary care for gender-diverse youth: a narrative review and unique model of gender-affirming care. Transgend Health. 2016;1(1):117–23. https://doi.org/10.1089/trgh.2016.0009.
14. Khatchadourian K, Amed S, Metzger DL. Clinical management of youth with gender dysphoria in Vancouver. J Pediatr. 2014;164(4):906–11. https://doi.org/10.1016/j.jpeds.2013.10.068.
15. Mahfouda S, Moore JK, Siafarikas A, Zepf FD, Lin A. Puberty suppression in transgender children and adolescents. Lancet Diabetes Endocrinol. 2017;5(10):816–26. https://doi.org/10.1016/S2213-8587(17)30099-2.
16. Bangalore Krishna K, Fuqua JS, Rogol AD, Klein KO, Popovic J, Houk CP, Charmandari E, et al. Use of gonadotropin-releasing hormone analogs in children: update by an international consortium. Horm Res Paediatr. 2019;91(6):357–72. https://doi.org/10.1159/000501336.
17. Rosenthal SM. Approach to the patient: transgender youth: endocrine considerations. J Clin Endocrinol Metab. 2014;99(12):4379–89. https://doi.org/10.1210/jc.2014-1919.
18. Todd NJ. At risk of pregnancy? Contraception for transgender, nonbinary, gender-diverse, and Two Spirit patients. BCMJ. 2022;64(2):69–74. Available from: https://bcmj.org/articles/risk-pregnancy-contraception-transgender-nonbinary-gender-diverse-and-two-spirit-patients. Accessed 9 May 2022
19. Mahfouda S, Moore JK, Siafarikas A, Hewitt T, Ganti U, Lin A, et al. Gender-affirming hormones and surgery in transgender children and adolescents. Lancet Diabetes Endocrinol. 2019;7(6):484–98. https://doi.org/10.1016/S2213-8587(18)30305-X.
20. Rafferty J, Committee On Psychosocial Aspects Of Child And Family Health; Committee On Adolescence; Section On Lesbian, Gay, Bisexual, And Transgender Health And Wellness. Ensuring comprehensive care and support for transgender and gender-diverse children and adolescents. Pediatrics. 2018;142(4):e20182162. https://doi.org/10.1542/peds.2018-2162.
21. Ehrensaft D. Gender nonconforming youth: current perspectives. Adolesc Health Med Ther. 2017;8:57–67. https://doi.org/10.2147/AHMT.S110859.

22. Hidalgo MA, Ehrensaft D, Tishelman AC, Clark LF, Garofalo R, Rosenthal SM, et al. The gender affirmative model: what we know and what we aim to learn. Hum Dev. 2013;56:285–90. https://doi.org/10.1159/000355235.
23. Quain KM, Kyweluk MA, Sajwani A, Gruschow S, Finlayson C, Gordon EJ, et al. Timing and delivery of fertility preservation information to transgender adolescents, young adults, and their parents. J Adolesc Health. 2021;68(3):619–22. https://doi.org/10.1016/j.jadohealth.2020.06.044.
24. Taylor AB, Chan A, Hall SL, Saewyc EM, the Canadian Trans & Non-binary Youth Health Survey Research Group. Being safe, being me 2019: results of the Canadian Trans and Non-binary Youth Health Survey. Vancouver, Canada: Stigma and Resilience Among Vulnerable Youth Centre, University of British Columbia; 2020. Available from: https://apsc-saravyc.sites.olt.ubc.ca/files/2020/12/Being-Safe-Being-Me-2019_SARAVYC_ENG_1.2.pdf. Accessed 22 Apr 2022
25. Grossman AH, D'Augelli AR. Transgender youth: invisible and vulnerable. J Homosex. 2006;51(1):111–28. https://doi.org/10.1300/J082v51n01_06.
26. James SE, Herman JL, Rankin S, Keisling M, Mottet L, Anafi M. The report of the 2015 U.S. Transgender Survey. Washington, DC: National Center for Transgender Equality; 2016. Available from: https://transequality.org/sites/default/files/docs/usts/USTS-Full-Report-Dec17.pdf. Accessed 22 Apr 2022
27. Waite S. Should I stay or should I go? Employment discrimination and workplace harassment against transgender and other minority employees in Canada's federal public service. J Homosex. 2021;68(11):1833–59. https://doi.org/10.1080/00918369.2020.1712140.
28. Flaskerud JH, Lesser J. The current socio-political climate and psychological distress among transgender people. Issues Ment Health Nurs. 2018;39(1):93–6.
29. Winter S, Diamond M, Green J, Karasic D, Reed T, Whittle S, et al. Transgender people: health at the margins of society. Lancet. 2016;388:390–400. https://doi.org/10.1016/S0140-6736(16)00683-8.
30. Reisner SL, Greytak EA, Parsons JT, Ybarra ML. Gender minority social stress in adolescence: disparities in adolescent bullying and substance use by gender identity. J Sex Res. 2015;52(3):243–56. https://doi.org/10.1080/00224499.2014.886321.
31. Heino E, Ellonen N, Kaltiala R. Transgender identity is associated with bullying involvement among finnish adolescents. Front Psychol. 2021;11:612424. https://doi.org/10.3389/fpsyg.2020.612424.
32. Clark TC, Lucassen MF, Bullen P, Denny SJ, Fleming TM, Robinson EM, et al. The health and well-being of transgender high school students: results from the New Zealand adolescent health survey (Youth'12). J Adolesc Health. 2014;55(1):93–9. https://doi.org/10.1016/j.jadohealth.2013.11.008.
33. Gonzales G, Deal C. Health risk factors and outcomes among gender minority high school students in 15 US States. JAMA. 2022;327(15):1498–500. https://doi.org/10.1001/jama.2022.3087.
34. Johns MM, Lowry R, Andrzejewski J, Barrios LC, Demissie Z, McManus T, et al. Transgender identity and experiences of violence victimization, substance use, suicide risk, and sexual risk behaviors among high school students—19 states and large urban school districts, 2017. MMWR Morb Mortal Wkly Rep. 2019;68(3):67–71. https://doi.org/10.15585/mmwr.mm6803a3.
35. Stutterheim SE, van Dijk M, Wang H, Jonas KJ. The worldwide burden of HIV in transgender individuals: an updated systematic review and meta-analysis. PLoS One. 2021;16(12):e0260063. https://doi.org/10.1371/journal.pone.0260063.
36. Becasen JS, Denard CL, Mullins MM, Higa DH, Sipe TA. Estimating the prevalence of HIV and sexual behaviors among the US transgender population: a systematic review and meta-analysis, 2006–2017. Am J Public Health. 2019;109(1):e1–8. https://doi.org/10.2105/AJPH.2018.304727.

37. Nunes-Moreno M, Buchanan C, Cole FS, Davis S, Dempsey A, Dowshen N, et al. Behavioral health diagnoses in youth with gender dysphoria compared with controls: a PEDSnet study. J Pediatr. 2022;241:147–53.e1. https://doi.org/10.1016/j.jpeds.2021.09.032.
38. Bauer GR, Pacaud D, Couch R, Metzger DL, Gale L, Gotovac S, Trans Youth CAN! Research Team, et al. Transgender youth referred to clinics for gender-affirming medical care in Canada. Pediatrics. 2021;148(5):e2020047266. https://doi.org/10.1542/peds.2020-047266.
39. Veale JF, Watson RJ, Peter T, Saewyc EM. Mental health disparities among Canadian transgender youth. J Adolesc Health. 2017;60(1):44–9. https://doi.org/10.1016/j.jadohealth.2016.09.014.
40. Marshall E, Claes L, Bouman WP, Witcomb GL, Arcelus J. Non-suicidal self-injury and suicidality in trans people: a systematic review of the literature. Int Rev Psychiatry. 2016;28(1):58–69. https://doi.org/10.3109/09540261.2015.1073143.
41. Diemer EW, White Hughto JM, Gordon AR, Guss C, Austin SB, Reisner SL. Beyond the binary: differences in eating disorder prevalence by gender identity in a transgender sample. Transgend Health. 2018;3(1):17–23. https://doi.org/10.1089/trgh.2017.0043.
42. Chodzen G, Hidalgo MA, Chen D, Garofalo R. Minority stress factors associated with depression and anxiety among transgender and gender-nonconforming youth. J Adolesc Health. 2019;64(4):467–71. https://doi.org/10.1016/j.jadohealth.2018.07.006.
43. Meyer IH. Prejudice as stress: conceptual and measurement problems. Am J Public Health. 2003;93(2):262–5. https://doi.org/10.2105/ajph.93.2.262.
44. Testa RJ, Michaels MS, Bliss W, Rogers ML, Balsam KF, Joiner T. Suicidal ideation in transgender people: gender minority stress and interpersonal theory factors. J Abnorm Psychol. 2017;126:125–36. https://doi.org/10.1037/abn0000234.
45. Tankersley AP, Grafsky EL, Dike J, Jones RT. Risk and resilience factors for mental health among transgender and gender nonconforming (TGNC) youth: a systematic review. Clin Child Fam Psychol Rev. 2021;24(2):183–206. https://doi.org/10.1007/s10567-021-00344-6.
46. Abramovich A, De Oliveira C, Kiran T, Iwajomo T, Ross LE, Kurdyak P. Assessment of health conditions and health service use among transgender patients in Canada. JAMA Netw Open. 2020;3:e2015036. https://doi.org/10.1001/jamanetworkopen.2020.15036.
47. Markovic L, McDermott D, Stefanac S, Seiler-Ramadas R, Iabloncsik D, Smith L, et al. Experiences and interactions with the healthcare system in transgender and non-binary patients in Austria: an exploratory cross-sectional study. Int J Environ Res Public Health. 2021;18:6895. https://doi.org/10.3390/ijerph18136895.
48. Goldberg AE, Kuvalanka KA, Budge SL, Benz MB, Smith JZ. Health care experiences of transgender binary and nonbinary university students. Couns Psychol. 2019;47:59–97. https://doi.org/10.1177/0011000019827568.
49. Clark BA, Veale JF, Greyson D, Saewyc E. Primary care access and foregone care: a survey of transgender adolescents and young adults. Fam Pract. 2018;35(3):302–6. https://doi.org/10.1093/fampra/cmx112.
50. Dowshen N, Lee S, Franklin J, Castillo M, Barg F. Access to medical and mental health services across the HIV care continuum among young transgender women: a qualitative study. Transgend Health. 2017;2(1):81–90. https://doi.org/10.1089/trgh.2016.0046.
51. Bauer GR, Hammond R, Travers R, Kaay M, Hohenadel KM, Boyce M. "I don't think this is theoretical; this is our lives": how erasure impacts health care for transgender people. J Assoc Nurses AIDS Care. 2009;20(5):348–61. https://doi.org/10.1016/j.jana.2009.07.004.
52. Ginsburg KR, Winn RJ, Rudy BJ, Crawford J, Zhao H, Schwarz DF. How to reach sexual minority youth in the health care setting: the teens offer guidance. J Adolesc Health. 2002;31(5):407–16. https://doi.org/10.1016/S1054-139X(02)00419-6.
53. Chong LSH, Kerklaan J, Clarke S, Kohn M, Baumgart A, Guha C, et al. Experiences and perspectives of transgender youths in accessing health care: a systematic review. JAMA Pediatr. 2021;175(11):1159–73. https://doi.org/10.1001/jama.

54. Olson KR, Durwood L, DeMeules M, McLaughlin KA. Mental health of transgender children who are supported in their identities. Pediatrics. 2016;137(3):e20153223. https://doi.org/10.1542/peds.2015-3223.
55. Russell ST, Pollitt AM, Li G, Grossman AH. Chosen name use is linked to reduced depressive symptoms, suicidal ideation, and suicidal behavior among transgender youth. J Adolesc Health. 2018;63(4):503–5. https://doi.org/10.1016/j.jadohealth.2018.02.003.
56. Pullen Sansfaçon A, Temple-Newhook J, Suerich-Gulick F, Feder S, Lawson ML, Ducharme J, et al. The experiences of gender diverse and trans children and youth considering and initiating medical interventions in Canadian gender-affirming speciality clinics. Int J Transgend. 2019;20:371–87. https://doi.org/10.1080/15532739.2019.1652129.
57. Connolly MD, Zervos MJ, Barone CJ 2nd, Johnson CC, Joseph CL. The mental health of transgender youth: advances in understanding. J Adolesc Health. 2016;59(5):489–95. https://doi.org/10.1016/j.jadohealth.2016.06.012.
58. Tordoff DM, Wanta JW, Collin A, Stepney C, Inwards-Breland DJ, Ahrens K. Mental health outcomes in transgender and nonbinary youths receiving gender-affirming care. JAMA Netw Open. 2022;5(2):e220978. https://doi.org/10.1001/jamanetworkopen.2022.0978.
59. van der Miesen AI, Steensma TD, de Vries AL, Bos H, Popma A. Psychological functioning in transgender adolescents before and after gender-affirmative care compared with cisgender general population peers. J Adolesc Health. 2020;66:699–704. https://doi.org/10.1016/j.jadohealth.2019.12.018.
60. De Vries AL, McGuire JK, Steensma T, Wagenaar ECF, Doreleijers TA, Cohen-Kettenis PT. Young adult psychological outcome after puberty suppression and gender reassignment. Pediatrics. 2014;134:696–704. https://doi.org/10.1542/peds.2013-2958.
61. de Vries AL, Steensma TD, Doreleijers TA, Cohen-Kettenis PT. Puberty suppression in adolescents with gender identity disorder: a prospective follow-up study. J Sex Med. 2011;8:2276–83.
62. Turban JL, King D, Carswell JM, Keuroghlian A. Pubertal suppression for transgender youth and risk of suicidal ideation. Pediatrics. 2020;145:e20191725. https://doi.org/10.1542/peds.2019-1725.
63. Kuper LE, Stewart S, Preston S, Lau M, Lopez X. Body dissatisfaction and mental health outcomes of youth on gender-affirming hormone therapy. Pediatrics. 2020;145(4):e20193006. https://doi.org/10.1542/peds.2019-3006.
64. Green AE, DeChants JP, Price MN, Davis CK. Association of gender-affirming hormone therapy with depression, thoughts of suicide, and attempted suicide among transgender and nonbinary youth. J Adolesc Health. 2021.:S1054-139X(21)00568-1; https://doi.org/10.1016/j.jadohealth.2021.10.036.
65. Seelman KL, Colón-Diaz MJP, LeCroix RH, Xavier-Brier M, Kattari L. Transgender non-inclusive healthcare and delaying care because of fear: connections to general health and mental health among transgender adults. Transgend Health. 2017;2(1):17–28. https://doi.org/10.1089/trgh.2016.0024.
66. Kreukels BP, Cohen-Kettenis PT. Puberty suppression in gender identity disorder: the Amsterdam experience. Nat Rev Endocrinol. 2011;7(8):466–72. https://doi.org/10.1038/nrendo.2011.78.
67. Cohen-Kettenis PT, Schagen SE, Steensma TD, de Vries AL, Delemarre-van de Waal HA. Puberty suppression in a gender-dysphoric adolescent: a 22-year follow-up. Arch Sex Behav. 2011;40(4):843–7.
68. Wood H, Sasaki S, Bradley SJ, Singh D, Fantus S, Owen-Anderson A, et al. Patterns of referral to a gender identity service for children and adolescents (1976–2011): age, sex ratio, and sexual orientation. J Sex Marital Ther. 2013;39:1–6. https://doi.org/10.1080/0092623X.2012.675022.

69. Wiepjes CM, Nota NM, de Blok CJM, Klaver M, de Vries ALC, Wensing-Kruger SA, et al. The Amsterdam cohort of gender dysphoria study (1972-2015): trends in prevalence, treatment, and regrets. J Sex Med. 2018;15(4):582–90. https://doi.org/10.1016/j.jsxm.2018.01.016.
70. Handler T, Hojilla JC, Varghese R, Wellenstein W, Satre DD, Zaritsky E. Trends in referrals to a pediatric transgender clinic. Pediatrics. 2019;144(5):e20191368. https://doi.org/10.1542/peds.2019-1368.
71. Gridley SJ, Crouch JM, Evans Y, Eng W, Antoon E, Lyapustina M, et al. Youth and caregiver perspectives on barriers to gender-affirming health care for transgender youth. J Adolesc Health. 2016;59(3):254–61. https://doi.org/10.1016/j.jadohealth.2016.03.017.
72. Safer JD, Coleman E, Feldman J, Garofalo R, Hembree W, Radix A, Sevelius J. Barriers to healthcare for transgender individuals. Curr Opin Endocrinol Diabetes Obes. 2016;23(2):168–71. https://doi.org/10.1097/MED.0000000000000227.
73. Sanchez NF, Sanchez JP, Danoff A. Health care utilization, barriers to care, and hormone usage among male-to-female transgender persons in New York City. Am J Public Health. 2009;99:713–9. https://doi.org/10.2105/AJPH.2007.132035.
74. Chan B, Skocylas R, Safer JD. Gaps in transgender medicine content identified among Canadian medical school curricula. Transgend Health. 2016;1(1):142–50.
75. Obedin-Maliver J, Goldsmith ES, Stewart L, White W, Tran E, Brenman S, Wells M, Fetterman DM, Garcia G, Lunn MR. Lesbian, gay, bisexual, and transgender–related content in undergraduate medical education. JAMA. 2011;306(9):971–7.
76. Vance SR Jr, Halpern-Felsher BL, Rosenthal SM. Health care providers' comfort with and barriers to care of transgender youth. J Adolesc Health. 2015;56(2):251–3. https://doi.org/10.1016/j.jadohealth.2014.11.002.
77. Dahlgren Allen S, Tollit MA, McDougall R, Eade D, Hoq M, Pang KC. A wait-list intervention for transgender young people and psychosocial outcomes. Pediatrics. 2021;148(2):e2020042762. https://doi.org/10.1542/peds.2020-042762.
78. Hamnvik OPR, Agarwal S, AhnAllen CG, Goldman AL, Reisner SL. Telemedicine and inequities in health care access: the example of transgender health Transgend Health 2020;7(2):113-116. doi: https://doi.org/10.1089/trgh.2020.0122
79. Hsieh S, Leininger J. Resource list: clinical care programs for gender-nonconforming children and adolescents. Pediatr Ann. 2014;43(6):238–44.
80. Silva C, Fung A, Irvine MA, Ziabakhsh S, Hursh BE. Usability of virtual visits for the routine clinical care of trans youth during the COVID-19 pandemic: youth and caregiver perspectives. Int J Environ Res Public Health. 2021;18(21):11321. https://doi.org/10.3390/ijerph182111321.
81. Jackson KJ, Tomlinson S. A review of top performing rural community and critical access hospitals' web resources for transgender patients in the United States. Sex Reprod Healthc. 2021;29:100627. https://doi.org/10.1016/j.srhc.2021.100627.
82. Gandy ME, Kidd KM, Weiss J, Leitch J, Hersom X. Trans*forming access and care in rural areas: a community-engaged approach. Int J Environ Res Public Health. 2021;18(23):12700. https://doi.org/10.3390/ijerph182312700.
83. Stroumsa D. The state of transgender health care: policy, law, and medical frameworks. Am J Public Health. 2014;104(3):e31–8. https://doi.org/10.2105/AJPH.2013.301789.
84. Kidd JD, Jackman KB, Barucco R, Dworkin JD, Dolezal C, Navalta TV, et al. Understanding the impact of the COVID-19 pandemic on the mental health of transgender and gender non-binary individuals engaged in a longitudinal cohort study. J Homosex. 2021;68(4):592–611. https://doi.org/10.1080/00918369.2020.1868185.
85. Guss CE, Woolverton GA, Borus J, Austin SB, Reisner SL, Katz-Wise SL. Transgender adolescents' experiences in primary care: a qualitative study. J Adolesc Health. 2019;65(3):344–9. https://doi.org/10.1016/j.jadohealth.2019.03.009.

86. Hedrick HR, Glover NT, Guerriero JT, Connelly KJ, Moyer DN. A new virtual reality: benefits and barriers to providing pediatric gender-affirming health care through telehealth. Transgend Health. 2022;7(2):144–9. https://doi.org/10.1089/trgh.2020.0159.
87. Stoehr JR, Jahromi AH, Hunter EL, Schechter LS. Telemedicine for gender-affirming medical and surgical care: a systematic review and call-to-action. Transgend Health. 2022;7(2):117–26. https://doi.org/10.1089/trgh.2020.0136.
88. Grasso C, Campbell J, Yunkun E, Todisco D, Thompson J, Gonzalez A, et al. Gender-affirming care without walls: utilization of telehealth services by transgender and gender diverse people at a federally qualified health center. Transgend Health. 2022;7(2):135–43. https://doi.org/10.1089/trgh.2020.0155.
89. Lock L, Anderson B, Hill BJ. Transgender care and the COVID-19 pandemic: exploring the initiation and continuation of transgender care in-person and through telehealth. Transgend Health. 2022;7(2):165–9. https://doi.org/10.1089/trgh.2020.01.
90. Gava G, Seracchioli R, Meriggiola MC. Telemedicine for endocrinological care of transgender subjects during COVID-19 pandemic. Evid Based Ment Health. 2020;23:e1. https://doi.org/10.1136/ebmental-2020-300201.
91. Sequeira GM, Kidd KM, Coulter RW, Miller E, Fortenberry D, Garofalo R, et al. Transgender youths' perspectives on telehealth for delivery of gender-affirming care. J Adolesc Health. 2020;68:1207–10. https://doi.org/10.1016/j.jadohealth.2020.08.028.
92. Committee on Pediatric Workforce, Marcin JP, Rimsza ME, Moskowitz WB. The use of telemedicine to address access and physician workforce shortages. Pediatrics. 2015;136(1):202–9. https://doi.org/10.1542/peds.2015-1253.
93. Sequeira GM, Kidd KM, Rankine J, Miller E, Ray KN, Fortenberry JD, et al. Gender-diverse youth's experiences and satisfaction with telemedicine for gender-affirming care during the COVID-19 pandemic. Transgend Health. 2022;7(2):127–34. https://doi.org/10.1089/trgh.2020.0148.
94. Roller CG, Sedlak C, Draucker CB. Navigating the system: how transgender individuals engage in health care services. J Nurs Scholarsh. 2015;47(5):417–24. https://doi.org/10.1111/jnu.12160.
95. Julian JM, Salvetti B, Held JI, Murray PM, Lara-Rojas L, Olson-Kennedy J. The impact of chest binding in transgender and gender diverse youth and young adults. J Adolesc Health. 2021;68(6):1129–34. https://doi.org/10.1016/j.jadohealth.2020.09.029.
96. Vardi Y, Wylie KR, Moser C, Assalian P, Dean J, Asscheman H. Is physical examination required before prescribing hormones to patients with gender dysphoria? J Sex Med. 2008;5(1):21–6. https://doi.org/10.1111/j.1743-6109.2007.00681.x.
97. Damian AJ, Stinchfield K, Kearney RT. Telehealth and beyond: promoting the mental well-being of children and adolescents during COVID. Front Pediatr. 2022;10:793167. https://doi.org/10.3389/fped.2022.793167.
98. Gotkiewicz D, Goldstein TR. Extending our virtual reach: pediatricians and mental health providers bridging the chasm to mental health care for adolescents and transition-age youth during COVID-19. Clin Pediatr (Phila). 2021;60(9-10):389–91. https://doi.org/10.1177/00099228211034644.
99. Apple DE, Lett E, Wood S, Baber KF, Chuo J, Schwartz LA, et al. Acceptability of telehealth for gender-affirming care in transgender and gender diverse youth and their caregivers. Transgend Health. 2022;7(2):159–64. https://doi.org/10.1089/trgh.2020.0166.
100. Fox DA, Tan M, Lalani R, Atkinson L, Hursh B, Metzger DL. Evaluating the impact of a new intake process for British Columbia Children's Hospital Gender Clinic. J Endocr Soc. 2020;4:MON-LB302. https://doi.org/10.1210/jendso/bvaa046.2158.
101. Pampati S, Andrzejewski J, Steiner RJ, Rasberry CN, Adkins SH, Lesesne CA, et al. "We deserve care and we deserve competent care": qualitative perspectives on health care from transgender youth in the Southeast United States. J Pediatr Nurs. 2021;56:54–9. https://doi.org/10.1016/j.pedn.2020.09.021.

102. Rush KL, Howlett L, Munro A, Burton L. Videoconference compared to telephone in healthcare delivery: a systematic review. Int J Med Inform. 2018;118:44–53. https://doi.org/10.1016/j.ijmedinf.2018.07.007.
103. Canadian Medical Association. Virtual care playbook for Canadian physicians. Ottawa (CA): CMA; 2021. Available from: https://www.cma.ca/sites/default/files/pdf/Virtual-Care-Playbook_mar2020_E.pdf. Accessed 9 May 2022
104. Hardcastle L, Ogbogu U. Virtual care: enhancing access or harming care? Healthc Manage Forum. 2020;33(6):288–92. https://doi.org/10.1177/0840470420938818.

Chapter 12
Telehealth for Adolescents in the Juvenile Justice System

Rachel Ghosh, Victor Hsiao, and Do-Quyen Pham

Provision of Health Services for Detained Youth

Juvenile detention is a locked facility in which youth are held while awaiting resolution of their case. Detention facilities are meant to be temporary, finite, and brief; the median stay for detained youth is between 26 and 36 days according to data from 2019 [1]. Detained youth have a constitutional right to medical and mental healthcare, yet services can vary widely due to lack of clearly defined federal standards and differences in state laws regarding healthcare for detained youth [2]. Two factors remain constant across facilities: detained youth are disproportionately from communities of color and have experienced significant adverse childhood events (ACEs) and trauma, leading up to their encounters with the juvenile justice system and detention [3, 4].

While the National Commission on Correctional Healthcare (NCCHC) published guidelines for health services for detained youth, accreditation by NCCHC is voluntary for detention facilities [5]. These guidelines are supported by the American Academy of Pediatrics (AAP), American Academy of Child and Adolescent

R. Ghosh
Adolescent Medicine, Department of Youth Services, Boston Children's Hospital,
Boston, MA, USA
e-mail: rachel.ghosh@childrens.harvard.edu

V. Hsiao
Department of Pediatrics, Seattle Children's Hospital, University of Washington,
Seattle, WA, USA
e-mail: victor.hsiao@seattlechildrens.org

D.-Q. Pham (✉)
School Health, Maternal and Child Health, Fairfax County Health Department,
Fairfax, VA, USA
e-mail: doquyen.pham@fairfaxcounty.gov

© The Author(s), under exclusive license to Springer Nature
Switzerland AG 2024
Y. N. Evans et al. (eds.), *Telemedicine for Adolescent and Young Adult Health
Care*, https://doi.org/10.1007/978-3-031-55760-6_12

175

Psychiatry (AACAP), American College of Obstetricians and Gynecologists (ACOG), and the American Public Health Association (APHA) and recommend that detained youth be screened for urgent medical and mental health needs within the first few hours of their detainment and receive a comprehensive physical exam along with a care plan within 1 week of detention [2, 6].

Many detained youth have not had previous access to necessary medical and mental health care for a myriad of reasons, including lack of insurance or documentation, being the child of an undocumented parent, not attending school, neglect, history of abuse, and mistrust of medical and mental health institutions [7, 8]. According to Gallagher and Dobrin in 2007, healthcare services inside detention facilities tend to be offered "ad hoc," rather than systematically [9]. Therefore, while urgent healthcare issues may be prioritized, preventative healthcare efforts may be deferred. One study showed that 75% of youth on probation did not receive any of the NCCHC recommended services [10]. Missed opportunities abound for some of the most vulnerable youth in our country.

Detention facilities may contract with local institutions, including their local public health brigade, or private, for-profit practices to provide youth with necessary services and care. Government-affiliated contractors and larger facilities caring for youth with longer lengths of stay often have more resources on site and tend to provide more thorough, preventative care to youth [9]. Consistent access to medical and mental health providers offers opportunities for more comprehensive care and increased opportunities to support services that can promote healthy development of youth. Telehealth can be an additional tool that can help enhance services, care coordination, and referrals for youth, especially those detained in facilities that lack consistent access to a broad array of on-site resources [11].

Utilization of Telehealth to Enhance Healthcare Services for Detained Youth

Case 1

A youth presents to a local juvenile detention facility several months after her release from a state juvenile rehabilitation facility. You are the nurse practitioner on site and call her down to the clinic for her initial assessment. You notice a limp and in-toeing of her left leg as the youth walks into the exam room. She reports the history of a motor vehicle accident (MVA) that occurred prior to previous detainment. She shares that she was evaluated in the emergency room at the time of the MVA and had X-rays that were reassuring; otherwise, she did not receive additional imaging or follow-up care. She reports limitations to ambulation, though is guarded and declines a thorough physical exam.

Over the following week, you call the youth to the clinic multiple times in an effort to build rapport and reassess her leg. By the end of the week, she shares that she previously participated in volleyball, basketball, and track, competitively. Since the MVA, she has not participated in any sports. She reports chronic pain to her left leg and allows you to examine it. You note muscular atrophy, poor weight bearing, and limited range of motion at multiple joints of the left leg. You recommend an orthopedic consultation and further imaging to be done off site at the community hospital. The youth declines the referral, stating that she has been experiencing chronic pain for several months. She feels frustrated that she was not referred at the time of the accident or by previous providers. She has lost trust in the healthcare system and refuses further interventions. You acknowledge her frustrations and offer to coordinate a telehealth visit with the orthopedics team so that you can join her. You share that you can help her convey important details of her accident and current condition and ensure that follow-up care can be coordinated through the facility. After hearing this, she consents to the referral. You share the plan, obtain consent from her guardian, and schedule a telehealth visit with the orthopedist.

Black and Latinx youth are disproportionately detained and have been systematically disenfranchised from access to support systems in their community that could have prevented their entry into the justice system [12]. On initial visit with healthcare providers in juvenile detention, youth may be guarded and hesitant to share past medical history or current concerns. Reasons may range from a lack of knowledge in navigating the healthcare system at their stage of development to fear of repercussions in sharing sensitive information while detained. It is imperative for providers to ensure confidentiality and inform youth that records of healthcare services during detainment are separate from and not shared with the court system. Once trust is built, efforts by healthcare providers in detention facilities to coordinate with primary care providers and subspecialists can enhance experiences for detained youth and promote better outcomes. Utilization of telehealth can help facilitate this process.

Case 1: Key Takeaway Points

- While every effort should be made to assess a youth upon admission, building rapport and trust can take time and require multiple interactions.
- Many youth may have limited understanding of the healthcare system or have experienced bias in previous interactions.
- Telehealth is a modality that allows a provider in detention to accompany youth on their health visit and help advocate for their needs when seeing community subspecialists, to improve health outcomes.

Case 2

You are a mental health therapist working at a local juvenile detention center. A behavioral code is called in Unit A. You arrive in the unit to see that JB, a typically calm and composed youth, is visibly upset and has set off the sprinklers in the unit, causing the area to flood. All youth there are subsequently moved to a different unit. Due to his actions, JB is placed on restoration status where he is separated from his peers until his behavior is regulated. You offer to meet with him separately.

You ask if anything has upset him. He states "no" and is unable to look you in the eye. You recall that he had his first off-site visit with a physical therapist that day to address his shoulder injury. You ask him how the visit went and if his shoulder is feeling better. JB becomes tearful and shares that he doesn't want to go back to the clinic.

Upon further probing, JB shares that on arrival to the clinic, he had to walk through a general waiting room where he saw other kids and their parents. One child took out their phone and took a picture of him. He felt embarrassed as he was in his detention uniform and shackles. Kids in the waiting room whispered and pointed at him. He did not want to be seen in the community that way again. The experience made him feel ashamed and he was unable to focus on his appointment. He states he doesn't remember much of what his physical therapist reviewed with him.

You thank him for sharing his experience and feelings with you. You ask permission to speak to his pediatrician in the facility and his physical therapist in the community. After hearing your concerns, the team coordinates future physical therapy visits via telehealth. The physical therapy team delivers materials to help facilitate JB's exercises. JB completes future visits via telehealth and his condition improves. The clinic also re-evaluates their layout and identifies an alternate entrance to promote privacy for youth and other patients who may benefit from more discreet movement into and out of the clinic.

Prior to the facilitation of an off-site visit for a detained youth, several factors must be taken into consideration. On-site resources vary across facilities. Given safety and security guidelines, off-site appointments are limited to services and procedures that cannot be rendered inside secure detention. Depending on a youth's projected length of stay, non-urgent services and procedures may be deferred until after discharge.

Partnership with local community providers and facilities can help improve experiences for youth and enhance safety and security prior to transport. Staff at a detention center may request permission to visit a local hospital or clinic to map out alternate entries and exits prior to a youth's visit to promote privacy for detained youth when accessing care in the community. When possible, appointments with providers and imaging and/or procedures may be scheduled on the same day to maximize efficiency and limit transportation barriers. Telehealth can be a useful option to facilitate appointments for detained youth if proper examination and therapy can be provided across this modality. The use of telehealth for detained youth allows them to access care in a more private space. If youth require supervision or support during telehealth visits, efforts should be made to identify staff that they trust such as their primary provider in the facility or other professionals properly trained in HIPAA guidelines.

Case 2: Key Takeaway Points

- Dysregulation is often a sign that a youth may be experiencing emotional distress. Providing a safe space for them to express their frustrations can help identify the root cause of the issue.
- When accessing care off site, youth are accompanied by detention officers, shackled, and remain in detention uniforms, which can draw unwanted attention to them.
- Assessing community facilities and working with them to set up alternative entrance and exits can provide some privacy for detained youth.
- Telehealth, if appropriate, can allow youth to connect with their off-site care teams while bypassing security measures that often cause distress and barriers for detained youth when accessing other health facilities.

Discharge Planning and Reentry

Case 3

AJ presents to clinic to discuss discharge planning. They share that their next court date is in 2 weeks and they are excited to return home on electronic home monitoring. They have a history of depression, sexual assault, post-traumatic stress disorder, and opioid use disorder. They presented to detention 2 months ago in withdrawal from fentanyl. This was their second detainment, and school attendance prior to that was sporadic. Despite efforts to refer them to outpatient substance use treatment during their previous admission, the youth and their family were unable to follow up. Their father works two jobs and their mother is often caring for their younger sibling with special needs.

During this admission, they were started on daily suboxone and substance use therapy for withdrawal and management of opioid use disorder. They have found the medication to be helpful and now have aspirations to finish school and become a teacher. While they wish to continue care for opioid use disorder, they express anxiety about having to transition their healthcare to a new team. They are also worried they may not remember to take a daily medication after they leave the facility, given potential distractions at home. They are afraid that frequent visits for substance use therapy will be challenging for their family as well.

As the social worker on the team, you share the option of referral to the community's mobile medical team for substance use management. AJ agrees to meeting them via telehealth prior to discharge and an appointment is set up. AJ agrees to their parents' involvement in substance use treatment, allowing their mother to join the visit as well. At the telehealth visit, AJ and their mother meet the team's physician who shares different medication options for opioid use disorder including a monthly intramuscular (IM) injection of naltrexone. AJ and their family feel this would be a good option, and the care team coordinates the first administration prior to discharge from the facility. This includes reactivation of their Medicaid insurance, which was suspended upon admission, and a prior authorization request for naltrexone IM. AJ also meets with the mobile medical team's substance use therapist. He delivers a cellphone the following week so that AJ can easily access providers once discharged from the facility. The mobile medical team coordinates therapy via telehealth which AJ is able to attend using their new cell phone. The team provides additional home visits for medical follow-up and medication administration. Six months later, you receive a card at your workplace from AJ. They share that despite having to repeat the 11th grade, they were able to attend school consistently this year and just passed their midterms. AJ is receiving ongoing care for substance use disorder and has not used opioids since discharge from the facility.

Case 3: Key Takeaway Points

- Justice-involved youth have often endured numerous traumatic experiences. They and their family members often are juggling multiple responsibilities with limited resources.
- A clearly outlined discharge plan with proper accommodations such as equipment to promote consistent communication with their medical teams can help facilitate a smooth discharge.
- Telehealth, if accessible, allows a youth's guardian to be present during their discharge planning, allows the youth and their family to establish a relationship with their community providers prior to discharge, allows families to overcome certain logistical barriers, enhances ongoing care after release, and promotes a more successful re-entry into their communities.

Current Framework of Discharge Planning

The topic of effective discharge planning for detained youth is one that is becoming more widely discussed in efforts to improve post-discharge outcomes and reduce recidivism rates. The recommendations and utilization of telehealth in discharge planning, however, is limited. The American Academy of Pediatrics (AAP) and Substance Abuse Mental Health Services Administration (SAMHSA) call for the creation of a transitional plan prior to releasing youth into the community [13, 14]. These plans include involving parents/guardians and ensuring access to safe housing, food, medical and behavioral health services, health insurance, and educational services (including necessary Internet access and equipment). Community clinics have also been established to support youth following release. For instance, the University of New Mexico ADOBE Program seeks to provide wrap-around service for local, recently incarcerated youth, including medical and mental health, legal advice, home navigators, and educational support [15]. Current transitional interventions for reentry youth are, however, inconclusive and contradictory in regard to their efficacy [16].

In adult incarceration systems, various models exist. Ohio's Medicaid Pre-Release Program pre-enrolls persons who are incarcerated into a Medicaid health plan 30–60 days before release and utilizes video calls to connect inmates with health risk factors to care coordinators that can help develop a transition plan that covers needed doctor appointments as well as social needs [17, 18]. These case managers are required to contact enrollees within the first 5 days following release from prison and send them a letter with contact information for case management and services after there have been three unsuccessful attempts. One major challenge arises from inmates not always having a known or stable address or phone number prior to release. Meanwhile, the Transitions Clinic Network (TCN) is a nationwide medical homes network for individuals recently released from incarceration with chronic health conditions [19]. Through community health centers in neighborhoods most impacted by incarceration and employing formerly incarcerated individuals to work as community health workers, TCN seeks to promote access to services and continuity of care, provides medical services that are both culturally sensitive and patient-centered, and partners with local reentry and social services organizations to address social determinants of health. Their work has been found to decrease the number of emergency department visits and likelihood of individuals returning to prison for parole or probation due to technical violations [20, 21].

Current Needs for and Uses of Telehealth in Discharge Planning

On discharge, youth are often released with a long "to-do" list, including going to court hearings, meeting with probation/parole staff, enrolling for and attending school, and receiving medical care and therapies. Families are not always available or equipped to help youth with these tasks. Inability to comply with certain action items can result in re-arrest and recidivism, whether as a direct result of failing to comply or the indirect eventual consequences of not following through with certain items. One study found that among previously incarcerated individuals who were age 24 or younger, re-arrest rates were 75.9% at 3 years and 84.1% at 5 years [22].

There is little literature discussing the use of telehealth to facilitate discharge and optimize post-discharge outcomes for these youth. Based on our experience and the literature written on related topics, below are recommendations for uses of telehealth in discharge planning.

Using Telehealth as a Tool to Enhance Discharge Planning

Connection to Community Resources: Reentry Services, Care Coordination, and Health Insurance

The AAP and SAMHSA have provided good frameworks for needs of incarcerated youth, including involving parents/guardians and ensuring access to safe housing, food, medical and behavioral health services, health insurance, and educational services [2, 14]. Using technology can greatly assist with connecting youth and their families with these services prior to discharge. This is especially true amid the COVID-19 pandemic, when many reentry services have been interrupted and some have turned to utilizing more online means to serve their clients [23].

In a qualitative interview study by Barnert et al., parents and providers have noted different factors that impact the success of reentry, such as parental understanding and involvement, youth motivation, returning to a positive environment, and coordination among care teams [24]. In this study, three leverage points were identified to be of the highest yield for change: transportation, provider reliability and continuity, and health insurance. Telehealth would be incredibly helpful in addressing these leverage points. The use of telehealth eliminates the challenge of transportation as long as the patient has access to the proper equipment and has internet access. In the Connecticut Men's Health Reentry Study, participants described the difficulty of scheduling appointments around other reentry priorities such as work, parole reporting, and family commitments and would prefer using emergency room services as they could be seen immediately [25]. Telehealth appointments may offer more flexibility that may better fit the needs of patients following discharge.

Prior to discharge, telehealth can also help youth establish care with a future primary care provider or subspeciality team. In Barnert et al.'s study, parents and providers emphasized the importance of "continuity and accountability" and explained that "many community providers were apathetic about this population" and "youths' fear of being negatively judged by providers for their justice-involvement or risky health behaviors… caused youth to avoid seeking care." [24] To build rapport, parents emphasized the "continuity and accountability of providers even just showing up for scheduled in-home appointments" while providers had varied views; some commented on the need for more compassion toward the youth, while others cited family disengagement as the cause for disconnect [24].

Working with youth and their families to reestablish health insurance should also be included in discharge planning to avoid lapses in medical care, therapies, and medication adherence. This is especially important because the law requires the suspension of Medicaid while youth are in detention but not re-establishment upon release. Additional resources in addition to telehealth, such as legal assistance and financial supports, should be explored and offered to support families that may have additional considerations, such as immigration status or co-pays they cannot afford.

Strengthening Family Relationships

Family support and conflict are interrelated concepts. However, when examined independently, it was found that increased family conflict among incarcerated youth has been associated with increased family violence post-release; on the other hand, family support did not have any association [26]. Exploring ways, such as using video calls to conduct family-based interventions, to reduce family conflict among youth while in detention may be important for helping reduce post-discharge violence. A qualitative study examined the perspectives of defense lawyers, clinicians, and education advocates on families' experiences with the juvenile justice system in Los Angeles and found that families often lacked resources and felt shamed, needed to be empowered, and could benefit from mental health education and support [27]. To ensure a smooth transfer of care from the juvenile detention system, it is important to consider opportunities to empower and support families from the moment the youth are detained to when they are eventually released. Telehealth can be used to balance safety while also promoting care coordination and support of guardians and important family or community members. Family-based interventions, such as multidimensional family therapy and multisystemic therapy, have been shown to have improved outcomes for detained youth as well as their siblings [28]. Telehealth can be a valuable asset when trying to start these interventions prior to release from detention, in hopes that they will be continued following discharge.

Ensure Access to Necessary Equipment

It is critical to ensure that youth have the necessary equipment and access to the Internet so that they can access services including telehealth and reentry services. Having a device (such as phone, tablet, or laptop), potentially a camera, respective charging cables, as well as a place to charge these devices is necessary. Having a stable Internet access may be difficult due to factors such as cost, homelessness, and living in a rural area. Even when equipment and Internet access are available, it is also necessary to have a safe, confidential space for an extended conversation, which can be a challenge if there are many individuals living in the same space as the youth or if stable housing is a concern. Partnership with schools and local, trusted locations such as libraries and faith-based facilities can help ensure that youth have access to technology and spaces that can promote telehealth follow-up [29, 30].

Using Mobile-Based Interventions: Texting and Social Media

Mobile-based interventions have been explored in various at-risk populations, showing that they are well-received, but data is limited with regard to whether the interventions lead to improved health outcomes and prevent recidivism. One study among youth in a substance abuse recovery program found that 70% of youth endorsed text messaging as a viable intervention method post-treatment and recommended certain qualities in the texts to avoid relapse: "positive appraisal (90%), lifestyle change tips (85%), motivational reinforcing (80%), coping advice (75%), confidence boosters (65%), inspiration encouragement (55%), and informational resources (50%)." [31]. A systematic review by Catalani et al. found that the use of mobile health technology has been found to be acceptable and feasible in supporting HIV treatment and prevention, with few studies showing that these tools can be used to improve linkage to care, retention in care, and antiretroviral treatment adherence [32]. The utilization of texting and various social media apps is an area worth further exploring when discussing the use of technology in supporting youth, especially given the increased use of these modes of communication and entertainment in this population. Recommendations that have been proposed in using mobile health among detained youth include standardizing tools across providers; considering the ethics such as confidentiality of utilizing electronic communication means; studying the impacts of mobile-based health on youth and their families; and using electronic messaging systems to send reminders for appointments and medication administration times, information about community resources, mindfulness and self-monitoring strategies, and copies of post-discharge forms and instructions for reference [33].

Conclusion

Care for youth involved in the juvenile justice system can be fragmented due to multiple factors including accessibility issues for underserved communities, varying models of care across juvenile justice systems, disruption of healthcare coverage, and lack of research in this patient population, due to numerous ethical and logistical challenges. There is continued need for additional evaluation into interventions that are not only well-received but also lead to measurable improved outcomes among justice-involved youth. While there is limited data pertaining to telehealth in the facilitation of healthcare services for justice-involved youth, its incorporation in different stages of care, including accessing subspeciality care, discharge planning, and community re-entry, can be a powerful tool to improve access for youth and their families. Further research can help care teams and families maximize its impact to enhance the wellbeing of youth involved in the justice system.

References

1. Justice N. Median days in placement since admission, by placement status, 1997–2019 [Internet]. Ojjdp.gov. 2022 [cited 7 August 2022]. Available from: https://www.ojjdp.gov/ojstatbb/corrections/qa08405.asp?qaDate=2019
2. Owen M, Wallace S, Alderman E, Chung R, Grubb L, Lee J, et al. Advocacy and collaborative health care for justice-involved youth. Pediatrics. 2020;146:1.
3. Evens C, Stoep A II. Risk factors for juvenile justice system referral among children in a public mental health system. J Behav Health Serv Res. 1997;24(4):443–55.
4. Baglivio MT, Epps N, Swartz K, Huq MS, Sheer A, Hardt NS. The prevalence of adverse childhood experiences (ACE) in the lives of juvenile offenders. J Juv Justice. 2014;3:2.
5. Juvenile Standards—National Commission on Correctional Health Care [Internet]. National Commission on Correctional Health Care. 2015 [cited 7 August 2022]. Available from: https://www.ncchc.org/juvenile-facilities/
6. Simonian M, John R. The primary care management for youth experiencing incarceration. J Nurse Pract. 2018;14(9):650–6.e3
7. Mmari K, Marshall B, Lantos H, Blum R. Who adolescents trust may impact their health: findings from Baltimore. J Urban Health. 2016;93(3):468–78.
8. Molleman T, Leeuw F. The influence of prison staff on inmate conditions: a multilevel approach to staff and inmate surveys. Eur J Crim Policy Res. 2011;18(2):217–33.
9. Gallagher C, Dobrin A. Can juvenile justice detention facilities meet the call of the American Academy of Pediatrics and National Commission on Correctional Health Care? A National analysis of current practices. Pediatrics. 2007;119(4):e991–e1001.
10. White C. Treatment services in the juvenile justice system: examining the use and funding of services by youth on probation. Youth Violence Juvenile Justice. 2017;17(1):62–87.
11. Fox K, Whitt A. Telemedicine can improve the health of youths in detention. J Telemed Telecare. 2008;14(6):275–6.
12. Tolou-Shams M, Bath E, McPhee J, Folk J, Porche M, Fortuna L. Juvenile Justice, technology and family separation: a call to prioritize access to family-based telehealth treatment for justice-involved adolescents' mental health and well-being. Front Digit Health. 2022;4:867366.
13. Responding to the needs of youth involved with the justice system during the COVID-19 pandemic [Internet]. Aap.org. 2020 [cited 7 August 2022]. Available from: https://www.aap.org/en/pages/2019-novel-coronavirus-covid-19-infections/clinical-guidance/responding-to-the-needs-of-youth-involved-with-the-justice-system%2D%2Dduring-the-covid-19-pandemic/
14. Double Jeopardy: COVID-19 and behavioral health disparities for Black and Latino Communities in the U.S. Substance Abuse Mental Health Services Administration. 2020. [cited 7 August 2022]. Available from https://www.samhsa.gov/sites/default/files/covid19-behavioral-health-disparities-black-latino-communities.pdf
15. ADOBE Program :: HSC Research | The University of New Mexico [Internet]. Hsc.unm.edu. 2022 [cited 7 August 2022]. Available from: https://hsc.unm.edu/research/research-centers/institute-for-resilience-health-and-justice/adobe.html
16. Kvamme L, Waaler P, Helland S, Kjøbli J. Review: striving for happily ever after—supportive interventions for youth leaving residential placement—a systematic review. Child Adolesc Mental Health. 2021;
17. Bringing health care to people leaving the criminal justice system through in-reach programs [Internet]. Commonwealthfund.org. 2022 [cited 7 August 2022].

Available from: https://www.commonwealthfund.org/publications/2020/aug/bringing-health-care-people-leaving-criminal-justice-system-through-reach

18. Ohio's medicaid pre-release enrollment program [Internet]. Urban Institute. 2017 [cited 7 August 2022]. Available from: https://www.urban.org/research/publication/ohios-medicaid-pre-release-enrollment-program

19. Transitions Clinic [Internet]. Transitionsclinic.org. 2022 [cited 7 August 2022]. Available from: https://transitionsclinic.org/

20. Wang E, Hong C, Shavit S, Sanders R, Kessell E, Kushel M. Engaging individuals recently released from prison into primary care: a randomized trial. Am J Public Health. 2012;102(9):e22–9.

21. Wang E, Lin H, Aminawung J, Busch S, Gallagher C, Maurer K, et al. Propensity-matched study of enhanced primary care on contact with the criminal justice system among individuals recently released from prison to New Haven. BMJ Open. 2019;9(5):e028097.

22. Durose MR, Cooper AD, Snyder HN. Recidivism of prisoners released in 30 states in 2005: patterns from 2005-2010. U.S. Department of Justice: 2014 [cited 7 August 2022]. Available at https://bjs.ojp.gov/content/pub/pdf/rprts05p0510.pdf

23. Cohen R. Reentry in the wake of COVID-19: service providers adapt but need more support to address community needs—CSG Justice Center [Internet]. CSG Justice Center. 2021 [cited 7 August 2022]. Available from: https://csgjusticecenter.org/2021/11/02/reentry-in-the-wake-of-covid-19-service-providers-adapt-but-need-more-support-to-address-community-needs/

24. Barnert E, Abrams L, Lopez N, Sun A, Tran J, Zima B, et al. Parent and provider perspectives on recently incarcerated youths' access to healthcare during community reentry. Child Youth Serv Rev. 2020;110:104804.

25. Health Care after Incarceration. National Institute of Corrections. 2018 [cited 7 August 2022]. Available from: https://nicic.gov/health-care-after-incarceration

26. Mowen T, Fisher B. Youth reentry from prison and family violence perpetration: the salience of family dynamics. J Fam Violence. 2019;36(1):51–62.

27. Amani B, Milburn N, Lopez S, Young-Brinn A, Castro L, Lee A, et al. Families and the juvenile justice system. Fam Community Health. 2018;41(1):55–63.

28. Wagner D, Borduin C, Sawyer A, Dopp A. Long-term prevention of criminality in siblings of serious and violent juvenile offenders: a 25-year follow-up to a randomized clinical trial of multisystemic therapy. J Consult Clin Psychol. 2014;82(3):492–9.

29. DeGuzman P, Siegfried Z, Leimkuhler M. Evaluation of rural public libraries to address telemedicine inequities. Public Health Nurs. 2020;37(5):806–11.

30. Shelton R, Hall M, Ford S, Cosby R. Telehealth in a Washington, DC African American Religious Community at the Onset of COVID-19: showcasing a virtual health ministry project. Soc Work Health Care. 2021;60(2):208–23.

31. Gonzales R, Douglas Anglin M, Glik D. Exploring the feasibility of text messaging to support substance abuse recovery among youth in treatment. Health Educ Res. 2013;29(1):13–22.

32. Catalani C, Philbrick W, Fraser H, Mechael, Israelski D. mHealth for HIV treatment & prevention: a systematic review of the literature. Open AIDS J. 2013;7(1):17–41.

33. Bath E, Tolou-Shams M, Farabee D. Mobile Health (mHealth): building the case for adapting emerging technologies for justice-involved youth. J Am Acad Child Adolesc Psychiatry. 2018;57(12):903–5.

Index